SARS, MERS and other Viral Lung Infections

Edited by
David S. Hui, Giovanni A. Rossi
and Sebastian L. Johnston

Editor in Chief
Robert Bals

This book is one in a series of *ERS Monographs*. Each individual issue provides a comprehensive overview of one specific clinical area of respiratory health, communicating information about the most advanced techniques and systems required for its investigation. It provides factual and useful scientific detail, drawing on specific case studies and looking into the diagnosis and management of individual patients. Previously published titles in this series are listed at the back of this *Monograph*.

ERS Monographs are available online at www.erspublications.com and print copies are available from www.ersbookshop.com

Continuing medical education (CME) credits are available through many issues of the *ERS Monograph*. Following evaluation, successful *Monographs* are accredited by the European Board for Accreditation in Pneumology (EBAP) for 5 CME credits. To earn CME credits, read the book of your choice (it is clearly indicated on the online table of contents whether CME credits are available) then complete the CME question form that is available at www.ers-education.org/e-learning/cme-tests.aspx

Managing Editor: Rachel White
European Respiratory Society, 442 Glossop Road, Sheffield, S10 2PX, UK
Tel: 44 114 2672860 | E-mail: Monograph@ersj.org.uk

Published by European Respiratory Society ©2016
June 2016
Print ISBN: 978-1-84984-069-9
Online ISBN: 978-1-84984-070-5
Print ISSN: 2312-508X
Online ISSN: 2312-5098
Printed by Latimer Trend and Company Limited, Plymouth, UK

C O P E
Member since 2009
JM04643
This journal is a member of and subscribes to the principles of the Committee on Publication Ethics

MIX
Paper from responsible sources
FSC® C013436
www.fsc.org

THOMSON REUTERS BOOK CITATION INDEX INDEXED

ERS | *monograph*

Contents

SARS, MERS and other Viral Lung Infections

Number 72
June 2016

Preface

Robert Bals

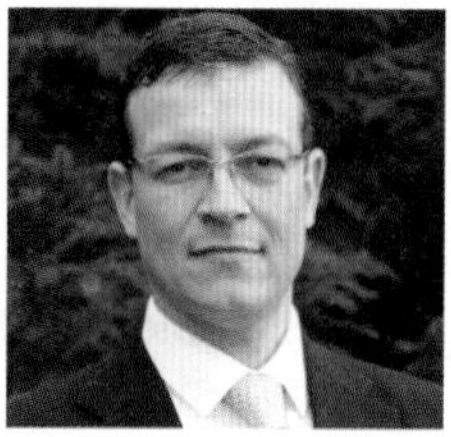

There is an ongoing debate whether viruses can be classified as life forms as they lack the characteristics (*e.g.* cell body or autarkic replication) of eukaryotic or prokaryotic cells. The emergence of viruses in evolutionary terms is also unclear; it is likely they have advanced from bacterial plasmids or other parts of nucleic acids. Virology was founded when Dmitri Ivanovsky and Martinus Beijerinck discovered plant viruses at the end of the 19th century. Viruses comprise complex particles that infect bacterial, plant and animal cells. They are classified by their genome (where ss is single stranded and ds is double stranded, according to the Baltimore classification) into dsDNA viruses, ssDNA viruses, dsRNA viruses, (+)ssRNA viruses, (−)ssRNA viruses, ssRNA-RT viruses and dsDNA-RT viruses. The classification of the International Committee on Taxonomy of Viruses (ICTV) divides virus by their biological properties into orders, families and so on. The morphologies of viruses are very diverse and comprise viruses with or without lipid cover and multiple shapes.

As the biological complexity of viruses unfolds, the pulmonary physician continues to face viral infections in daily practice: 1) typical respiratory viruses, such as influenza, rhinovirus or RSV, which cause common infectious diseases; 2) new viruses, which often originate in animals, become a threat to mankind and cause outbreaks (SARS-CoV and MERS-CoV); 3) immunocompromised patients who are susceptible to a wide range of viral species (CMV and herpes simplex virus); and 4) respiratory viruses and newly identified viruses, which have been shown to impact on the development of non-communicable diseases, such as asthma, COPD and perhaps cancer. Viral infections therefore play an important role in respiratory medicine and are within the main focus of public health activities.

This *ERS Monograph* considers viral infections of the respiratory tract with a focus on newly emerged viruses. There are chapters on SARS-CoV, MERS-CoV and avian influenza, as well as more common viral pathogens, such as seasonal influenza and rhinovirus.

 Print ISBN: 978-1-84984-069-9. Online ISBN: 978-1-84984-070-5. Print ISSN: 2312-508X. Online ISSN: 2312-5098.

The chapters present comprehensive information about the biology, diagnosis and treatment of the disease, and are written by experts in the field of world renown.

The European Respiratory Society is a partner of the Platform for European Preparedness Against (Re-)emerging Epidemics (PREPARE) (http://www.prepare-europe.eu), which is funded by the European Commission's 7th Framework Programme for Research and Technological Development (FP7) project. PREPARE aims to harmonise large-scale clinical research studies on infectious diseases, and is prepared to respond to severe infectious disease outbreak rapidly, in order to provide real-time evidence for clinical patient management and inform public health responses. PREPARE is a driving force in this area: it has already launched a range of interventional and observational interpandemic trials, and is working to reduce logistical, regulatory and administrative bottlenecks to speed the rapid implementation of clinical trials. With this initiative in mind, an *ERS Monograph* on viral diseases is very well timed.

The Guest Editors, David S. Hui, Giovanni A. Rossi and Sebastian L. Johnston have worked very successfully to integrate the selected topics into a comprehensive book that presents the current knowledge on viral infection. I would like to thank the Guest Editors and all the authors for their work on this excellent book. I am sure that this comprehensive review will be useful for the clinical practice of a broad range of respiratory physicians.

Disclosures: R. Bals has received grants from the German Research Ministerium and the Deutsche Forschungsgemeinschaft. He has also received personal fees from GSK, AstraZeneca, Boehringer Ingelheim and CSL Behrig.

Guest Editors

David S. Hui

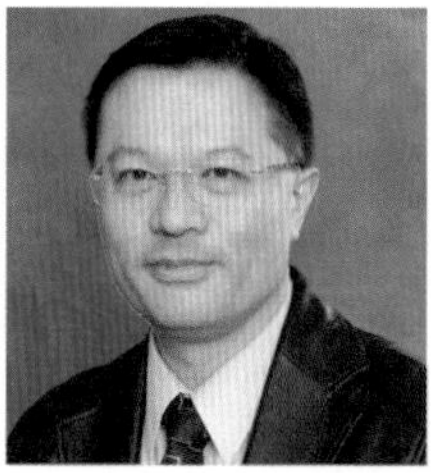

David S. Hui is the Stanley Ho Professor of Respiratory Medicine and Director of the Stanley Ho Centre for Emerging Infections Diseases at the Chinese University of Hong Kong (Shatin, Hong Kong).

He graduated from the University of New South Wales (Kensington, Australia) in 1985. He then trained in respiratory medicine and sleep medicine in Sydney, Australia. He was heavily involved in the clinical management of patients with SARS at the Prince of Wales Hospital (Shatin, Hong Kong) during the major outbreak in 2003. He served as a World Health Organization (WHO) advisor, reviewing the clinical management of avian influenza A(H5N1) during the early human outbreak in Vietnam in February 2004, and has since been a regular advisor to the WHO on the clinical management of SARIs. He has contributed to WHO treatment guidelines (including those for the influenza A(H5N1) virus in 2007, the influenza A(H1N1) pandemic in 2009, and MERS in 2013) and the WHO training workshop on the clinical management of influenza A(H7N9) and other SARIs in May 2014. He was a member of the urgent WHO missions investigating the outbreaks of MERS in Saudi Arabia and South Korea in 2013 and 2015, respectively.

David Hui's research interests include the clinical management of emerging SARIs, the safety of respiratory therapy in the post-SARS era, the efficacy of medical ward airflow in preventing nosocomial infections, sleep disordered breathing, and common airway diseases.

Giovanni A. Rossi

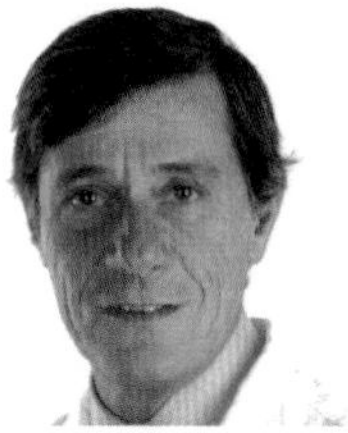

Giovanni A. Rossi is the former chief of the Pulmonary and Allergy units and of the Cystic Fibrosis Centre at the G. Gaslini Research Institute and University Hospital (Genoa, Italy) and the former adjunct Professor of Paediatric Pulmonology at the University of Genoa (Genoa). He is now Chief Emeritus at the G. Gaslini Research Institute.

 Print ISBN: 978-1-84984-069-9. Online ISBN: 978-1-84984-070-5. Print ISSN: 2312-508X. Online ISSN: 2312-5098.

Giovanni Rossi was Head of the Lung Cell Biology Assembly and a member of the Executive Committee of the European Respiratory Society, of which he has recently been appointed Foundation Fellow. He also served as an associate editor on the editorial boards of several other respiratory, allergy and paediatric journals and has published >290 manuscripts in peer reviewed journals.

His major areas of basic and clinical research have been the mechanisms involved in the pathogenesis of a variety of respiratory disorders, including the interstitial, obstructive and infectious diseases. In the latter, his work has focused mainly on the characterisation of the host–virus interaction at the lower respiratory tract level, with the aim of developing novel strategies for the prevention and treatment of these high-impact respiratory disorders for which specific therapies are often not yet available.

Sebastian L. Johnston

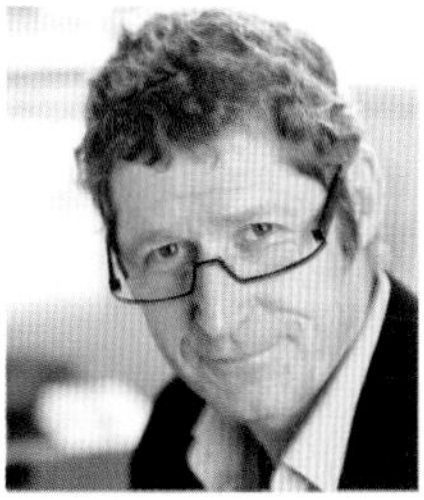

Sebastian L. Johnston is Professor of Respiratory Medicine and Allergy at the National Heart and Lung Institute, Imperial College London (London, UK). He is Director of the MRC and Asthma UK Centre in Allergic Mechanisms of Asthma (London), is the Asthma UK Clinical Professor and is a former European Research Council Advanced Grant holder. He is also a UK National Institute of Health Research Senior Investigator.

Sebastian Johnston edited *Thorax* from 2002 to 2010 and serves as an associate editor on the editorial boards of several other respiratory and allergy journals. He has published >380 scholarly manuscripts in peer reviewed journals and has 18 patents.

Notable discoveries that have emerged from his work include establishing the viral aetiology of the majority of asthma and COPD exacerbations, discovering novel mechanisms of susceptibility to virus infection in asthma and COPD, and developing novel treatment approaches for acute exacerbations of these diseases.

Sebastian Johnston is committed to capacity building for academia, industry and health services by training new basic and clinical investigators in asthma and COPD research. He also plays a significant role in public engagement and communication in the public domain.

ERS | *monograph*

Introduction

David S. Hui[1,2], Giovanni A. Rossi[3] and Sebastian L. Johnston[4]

Viral respiratory tract infections are important and common causes of morbidity and mortality worldwide. Over the past two decades, several novel viral respiratory infections with epidemic potential that threaten global health security have emerged. Human cases of the highly pathogenic avian influenza A(H5N1) were initially detected in Hong Kong in 1997, before spreading to other parts of Asia, the Middle East, Europe and Africa, with a case fatality rate close to 60%. Influenza A(H1N1)pdm09 virus first emerged in 2009 as a novel swine-origin strain, which rapidly led to a pandemic and has remained a common circulating strain in many parts of the world. Human infections with the novel avian influenza A(H7N9) virus were first reported in mainland China in March 2013 and the infection has since spread to Hong Kong and Taiwan. Avian influenza A(H5N1) and A(H7N9) viruses have continued to circulate widely in some poultry populations and infect humans sporadically; sporadic human cases of avian A(H5N6), A(H10N8) and A(H6N1) have also emerged.

In March 2003, the World Health Organization (WHO) issued a global alert about an emerging SARS caused by a novel CoV, which rapidly spread from mainland China *via* Hong Kong to at least 29 countries/regions and finally ended in July 2003, with 8096 probable cases and 774 deaths. Since its first discovery in a patient who died of severe pneumonia in Saudi Arabia in 2012, MERS-CoV has spread to 26 countries. The mortality rates of MERS-CoV infection are high, especially in those with comorbid disease.

In addition to the threat of novel CoV and avian influenza viruses, the burden of the common respiratory viruses, such as seasonal influenza, RSV and human rhinoviruses (HRV), on healthcare utilisation remains high, and yet is also a largely unmet medical need. This highlights the urgent need for developing more effective therapies in order to reduce the morbidity and mortality associated with novel threats, as well as the regular offenders.

The Platform for European Preparedness Against (Re-)emerging Epidemics (PREPARE) (http://www.prepare-europe.eu/) is an European Union funded network aiming to harmonise large-scale clinical research studies on infectious diseases, and provide real-time evidence for clinical management of patients and for informing public health responses. To advance our understanding of the clinical, epidemiological and scientific aspects of important respiratory viruses and facilitate planning of research studies on emerging

[1]Dept of Medicine and Therapeutics, The Chinese University of Hong Kong, Prince of Wales Hospital, Shatin, Hong Kong. [2]Stanley Ho Center for Emerging Infectious Disease, The Chinese University of Hong Kong, Prince of Wales Hospital, Shatin, Hong Kong. [3]Dept of Pediatrics, Pulmonary and Allergy Disease Units, Istituto G. Gaslini, Genoa, Italy. [4]National Heart & Lung Institute, Imperial College London, London, UK.

Correspondence: David S. Hui, Dept of Medicine, Chinese University of Hong Kong, Prince of Wales Hospital, Shatin, Hong Kong. E-mail: dschui@cuhk.edu.hk

 Print ISBN: 978-1-84984-069-9. Online ISBN: 978-1-84984-070-5. Print ISSN: 2312-508X. Online ISSN: 2312-5098.

infectious diseases, this *ERS Monograph* aims to provide an up-to-date and comprehensive overview of SARS, MERS and other viral respiratory infections, including seasonal influenza, avian influenza, RSV and HRV through six chapters written by authoritative experts from around the globe. We are most grateful to all the authors for their enormous contribution to this excellent book. We believe the selected topics will be of immense interest to all clinicians and scientists in the field.

Disclosures: S.L. Johnston reports receiving grants and personal fees from Centocor, Sanofi Pasteur, GSK, Chiesi, Boehringer Ingelheim and Novartis. He has also received personal fees from Grünenthal. He has received grants, personal fees and holds shares in Synairgen. In addition, S.L. Johnston has the following licensed patents. Blair ED, Killington RA, Rowlands DJ, Clarke NJ, Johnston SL. Transgenic animal models of HRV with human ICAM-1 sequences. UK patent application no. 02 167 29.4, 18 July 2002 and International patent application No. PCT/EP2003/007939, 17 July 2003; Wark PA, Johnston SL, Holgate ST, Davies DE. Anti-virus therapy for respiratory diseases. UK patent application no. GB 0405634.7, 12 March 2004; Wark PA, Johnston SL, Holgate ST, Davies DE. Interferon-beta for anti-virus therapy for respiratory diseases. International patent application no. PCT/GB05/50031, 12 March 2004; Wark PA, Johnston SL, Holgate ST, Davies DE. The use of interferon lambda for the treatment and prevention of virally-induced exacerbation in asthma and chronic pulmonary obstructive disease. UK patent application no. 0518425.4, 9 September 2005; Wark PA, Johnston SL, Holgate ST, Davies DE. Anti-virus therapy for respiratory diseases. US patent application - 11/517,763, patent no. 7569216, national phase of PCT/GB2005/050031, 04 August 2009; Wark PA, Johnston SL, Holgate ST, Davies DE. Interferon-beta for anti-virus therapy for respiratory diseases. European patent number 1734987, 5 May 2010; Wark PA, Johnston SL, Holgate ST, Davies DE. Anti-virus therapy for respiratory diseases (IFNb therapy) Hong Kong patent number 1097181, 31 August 2010; Wark PA, Johnston SL, Holgate ST, Davies DE. Anti-virus therapy for respiratory diseases (IFNb therapy). Japanese patent number 4807526, 26 August 2011; Wark PA, Johnston SL, Holgate ST, Davies DE. Interferon-beta for anti-Virus therapy for respiratory dseases. New Hong Kong - Divisional patent application no. 11100187.0, 10 January 2011. S.L. Johnston also has the following patent pending. Burdin N, Almond J, Lecouturieir V, Girerd-Chambaz Y, Guy B, Bartlett N, Walton R, McLean G, Glanville N, Johnston SL. Induction of cross-reactive cellular response against rhinovirus antigens. European Patent Number 13305152, 4 April 2013.

List of abbreviations

ARDS	acute respiratory distress syndrome
ARI	acute respiratory infection
BOOP	bronchiolitis obliterans organising pneumonia
CMV	cytomegalovirus
COP	cryptogenic organising pneumonia
COPD	chronic obstructive pulmonary disease
CoV	coronavirus
ICU	intensive care unit
IFN	interferon
Ig	immunoglobulin
IL	interleukin
ILI	influenza-like illness
MCP	monocyte chemoattractant protein
MERS	Middle East respiratory syndrome
RCT	randomised controlled trial
RSV	respiratory syncytial virus
RT-PCR	reverse transcriptase polymerase chain reaction
SARI	severe acute respiratory infection
SARS	severe acute respiratory syndrome
TLR	Toll-like receptors
TNF	tumour necrosis factor

Chapter 1

Severe acute respiratory syndrome coronavirus

David S. Hui[1,2] and Nelson Lee[1,2]

SARS, caused by a novel CoV, first emerged in Southern China in November 2002 before spreading to 29 countries/regions within a few weeks in 2003. Bats are natural reservoirs of SARS-like CoVs. The presence of SARS-like CoVs in horseshoe bats raised the possible role of bats in previous and future SARS outbreaks in humans. Tracheal intubation, manual ventilation before intubation, tracheotomy and noninvasive ventilation increased the risk of nosocomial SARS transmission to healthcare workers; a bed distance of <1 m apart, staff working while experiencing symptoms and high flow oxygen >6 L·min^{-1} increased the risk of super-spreading events. The unexpected emergence, rapid spread and high morbidity and mortality of SARS made it impossible to set up RCT of any antiviral agents and other therapies against SARS-CoV infection. Retrospective analyses of non-RCT data suggested that protease inhibitors, IFN and convalescent plasma might have some beneficial effects, whereas ribavirin led to significant haemolysis without any clinical benefit.

SARS-CoV first emerged in November 2002 in Southern China. During the global outbreak in 2003, mainland China [1], Hong Kong [2], Taiwan [3], Vietnam [4], Toronto (ON, Canada) [5] and Singapore [6] were the more severely affected countries/cities. The SARS-CoV epidemic involved 29 countries/regions and finally ended in July 2003, with 8096 probable cases of SARS-CoV infection and 774 deaths [7]. SARS-CoV infection posed an enormous public health threat and a major challenge to international health, in addition to having an adverse economic impact in the affected areas through disruption of business, social activities and air travel around the world [8].

Virology

CoVs (order *Nidovirales,* family *Coronaviridae*, subfamily *Coronavirinae*) are a group of single-stranded, enveloped, highly diverse, positive-sense, RNA viruses that may cause respiratory, hepatic, enteric and neurological diseases of varying severity in a wide range of animal species, including humans. CoVs are further divided into four genera: αCoV, βCoV, γCoV and δCoV [9]. A novel group 2b βCoV was discovered and confirmed in March 2003

[1]Dept of Medicine and Therapeutics, The Chinese University of Hong Kong, Prince of Wales Hospital, Shatin, Hong Kong. [2]Stanley Ho Center for Emerging Infectious Diseases, The Chinese University of Hong Kong, Prince of Wales Hospital, Shatin, Hong Kong.

Correspondence: David S. Hui, Dept of Medicine and Therapeutics, The Chinese University of Hong Kong, Shatin, New Territories, Hong Kong. E-mail: dschui@cuhk.edu.hk

 Print ISBN: 978-1-84984-069-9. Online ISBN: 978-1-84984-070-5. Print ISSN: 2312-508X. Online ISSN: 2312-5098.

as the causative agent responsible for SARS-CoV infection [10–12]. The genome sequence of the SARS-CoV was not closely related to any of the previously characterised CoVs [13–15].

The SARS-CoV genome contains 5′-methylated caps and 3′-polyadenylated tails and is arranged in the order of 5′, replicase genes, genes encoding structural proteins (spike glycoprotein (S), envelope protein (E), membrane protein (M) and nucleocapsid protein (N)), polyadenylated tail and then the 3′ end. The partially overlapping 5′-terminal open reading frame 1a/b is within the 5′ two-thirds of the CoV genome and encodes the large replicase polyprotein 1a (pp1a) and pp1ab. These polyproteins are cleaved by papain-like cysteine protease and 3C-like serine protease to produce nonstructural proteins, including RNA-dependent RNA polymerase and helicase, which are important enzymes involved in the transcription and replication of CoVs. The 3′ third of the CoV genome encodes the structural proteins (S, E, M and N), which are essential for virus–cell-receptor binding and virion assembly, and other nonstructural proteins and accessory proteins that may have immunomodulatory effects [9].

Host and reservoir

A high sero-prevalence (16.7%) was observed among asymptomatic wild animal salesmen in a retrospective serology study in Guangzhou in southern China. The data suggested that SARS-CoV infection might have transmitted from animal species to humans in a wet market [16]. In an animal market located in Shenzhen, a highly similar variant of SARS-CoV was detected in palm civets [17]. Masked palm civets were thus thought to be responsible for the transmission of SARS-CoV to humans because 30% of wild animal handlers were found to have positive serology against SARS-CoV infection compared to 1% of controls in the Guangdong province [17]. Furthermore, up to 39% of SARS-CoV cases that occurred in the early stage of the outbreak were associated with a history of exposure to animal markets [18]. Three of the four patients had indirect or direct contact with palm civets during the sporadic outbreaks of SARS-CoV infection in Guangzhou in December 2003 and January 2004 [19, 20]. Nevertheless, subsequent analysis of the viral genomic sequence revealed that the SARS-CoV-like virus had not been present for a long period among masked civet cats in markets. Instead, CoVs similar to SARS-CoV were detected in 2005 in Chinese horseshoe bats [21, 22]. These SARS-like CoVs from bats shared a high degree of sequence similarity (88–92%) with human or civet cat isolates, suggesting that bats could well be the natural source of an early ancestor of SARS-CoV [23]. It remains uncertain whether an intermediate mammalian host is involved prior to human transmission.

Pathogenesis

The respiratory tract is the entry site for SARS-CoV in humans; it is uncertain whether the gastrointestinal tract could be another entry route [24]. SARS-CoV infection occurs through a three-step process: receptor binding; induced conformational changes in S glycoprotein; cathepsin L proteolysis within endosomes [25]. Angiotensin-converting enzyme 2 (ACE2), a metallopeptidase which is expressed on a wide variety of human organ tissues, is the host functional receptor mediating the entry of SARS-CoV [26]. ACE2 is present in the epithelia of the human lungs and small intestine abundantly, and these might provide possible entry sites for SARS-CoV [27]. However, the presence of ACE2 might not be the only requirement for SARS-CoV tropism. For example, SARS-CoV was not detected in vascular endothelial cells and intestinal smooth muscle cells despite their abundant expression of ACE2, whereas SARS-CoV was found in colonic enterocytes and hepatocytes without ACE2 expression [27, 28]. The human C-type lectin was initially implicated as an alternative receptor in a cohort study of patients with SARS-CoV infection [29], but the observation could not be reproduced in two other studies [30, 31].

ACE2 may contribute to the development of diffuse alveolar damage (DAD). ACE2 is a negative regulator of the renin-angiotensin system by inactivating angiotensin II. SARS-CoV infections and the S glycoprotein of SARS-CoV could reduce ACE2 expression, whereas injection of SARS-CoV S glycoprotein into mice worsened acute lung injury *in vivo*, which could be reduced by blocking the renin-angiotensin pathway [32]. In addition, overexpression of SARS-CoV proteins, such as 3a and 7a proteins, expressed in the lungs and intestinal tissues of patients with SARS-CoV infection, could induce apoptosis *in vitro* [33, 34].

Lung histopathology features in patients with severe SARS-CoV infection included DAD, denudation of bronchial epithelia, loss of cilia, squamous metaplasia and giant-cell infiltrate, with a marked increase in macrophages in the alveoli and the interstitium. Haemophagocytosis, atrophy of the white pulp of the spleen, hyaline membranes and secondary bacterial pneumonia were also noted [2, 11, 35, 36]. While DAD was the main pulmonary feature [2, 11, 35], lesions in subpleural locations resembling COP were also seen [37]. In cynomologus macaques experimentally infected with SARS-CoV, extensive expression of SARS-CoV antigen in type I pneumocytes was noted early at day 4, suggesting that this cell type might be the primary target for SARS-CoV infection early in the disease [38].

Diarrhoea was reported by a quarter of patients with SARS-CoV infection [28, 39]. There were features of active viral replication within the small and large bowel in the presence of minimal architectural disruption in specimens obtained by *post mortem* examination or colonoscopy. Viral culture of these specimens confirmed SARS-CoV infection, whereas SARS-CoV RNA was positive in the stool specimens for almost 2.5 months after illness onset [28]. A higher mean nasopharyngeal SARS-CoV viral load on day 10 after illness onset had significant association with the presence of diarrhoea (3.1 *versus* 1.8 $\log_{10}$ copies·mL^{-1}; p=0.01) and mortality (6.2 *versus* 1.7 $\log_{10}$ copies·mL^{-1}; p<0.01) [40].

Activation of T-helper (Th1) cell-mediated immunity and hyper innate inflammatory response might be responsible for disease progression in SARS-CoV infection [35, 39]. In an uncontrolled study of 20 adults with SARS-CoV infection, marked increases in the levels of the Th1 inflammatory cytokines (IFN-γ, IL-1, IL-6 and IL-12) were noted for over 14 days after illness onset [41]. There were marked increases in chemokines, such as Th1 chemokine IFN-γ-inducible protein-10 (IP-10), neutrophil chemokine IL-8 and MCP-1 (MCP-1) [41]. In mice infected with SARS-CoV, T-cells played an important role in SARS-CoV clearance, whereas a reduced T-cell response contributed to severe disease [42]. In another study of mice infected with SARS-CoV, robust virus replication accompanied by delayed type I IFN (IFN-I) signalling was observed orchestrating inflammatory responses and lung immunopathology with reduced survival. IFN-I could be detected until after peaking of virus titres, but early administration of IFN-I ameliorated immunopathology. This delayed IFN-I signalling was thought to promote the accumulation of pathogenic inflammatory monocyte macrophages (IMMs), leading to elevated lung cytokine/chemokine levels, vascular leakage and impaired virus-specific T-cell responses, whereas genetic ablation of the IFN-αβ receptor or IMM depletion protected mice from fatal infection, without affecting viral load [43].

Furthermore, a study on the innate responses showed that TLR signalling through the TRIF adaptor protein might play a role in protecting mice from lethal SARS-CoV disease [44].

TLR3(−/−), TLR4(−/−), and TRAM(−/−) mice were found to be more susceptible to SARS-CoV than wild-type mice, although there was only transient weight loss without mortality. In contrast, mice deficient in the TLR3/TLR4 adaptor TRIF were highly susceptible to SARS-CoV infection, with marked weight loss, increased lung pathology, higher viral titres, reduced lung function and increased mortality. In TRIF(−/−) mice infected with SARS-CoV, distinct alterations in inflammation were present, including excess infiltration of neutrophils and inflammatory cell types that correlated with increased pathology of other known causes of ARDS. Aberrant pro-inflammatory cytokine, chemokine and IFN-stimulated gene signalling programmes were also observed following infection of TRIF(−/−) mice that were similar to those seen in human patients with poor disease outcome following SARS-CoV infection. These findings highlight the importance of TLR receptor signalling in generating a balanced protective innate immune response to highly pathogenic CoV infections [44]. In addition, SARS-CoV M protein may function as a cytosolic pathogen-associated molecular pattern that stimulates IFN-β production by activating a TLR-related TNF receptor-associated factor 3-independent signalling cascade [45].

A case–control study conducted in Chinese patients with SARS-CoV infection and healthy controls has shown that genetic variants of IL-12 receptor B1 predispose to SARS-CoV infection, but are not necessarily associated with disease progression [46]. Another case–control study has shown that Mannose-binding lectin (MBL), a key molecule in innate immunity that functions as an ante-antibody before specific antibody response, contributes to the first-line host defense against SARS-CoV and that MBL deficiency is a susceptibility factor for acquisition of SARS-CoV infection [47].

Epidemiology and disease transmission

Guangdong province in southern China was the first place in which cases of SARS-CoV infection had occurred early. In November 2002, an outbreak of "atypical pneumonia" of uncertain aetiology occurred in Foshan; many healthcare workers became infected [48]. A retrospective study of 55 patients hospitalised with atypical pneumonia between 24 January 2003 and 18 February 2003 was performed in a Guangzhou city hospital. The study showed that three patients had a positive culture of SARS-CoV in their nasopharyngeal aspirates, while 48 (87%) showed positive serology to SARS-CoV in the convalescent period. Analysis of the genetic sequence of the virus isolated from patients in Guangdong showed that it was the prototype of the SARS-CoV found in other regions and countries [49].

A 64-year-old male renal physician who travelled from the Guangdong province on 21 February 2003 to attend a wedding dinner in Hong Kong, was the index case of the major SARS-CoV outbreak in Hong Kong [2, 5, 6, 50]. At least 16 hotel guests/visitors acquired SARS-CoV infection while they were visiting friends or staying on the same hotel floor as the Guangdong physician, who subsequently died of severe pneumonia a few days later at a hospital near the hotel [35]. Owing to the swiftness of international air travel, SARS-CoV infection was spread to 29 countries/regions within a few weeks by these hotel guests [1, 51]. SARS-CoV seems to spread predominantly by close contact with an infected person through transmission of respiratory droplets or contact with fomite [52]. The nosocomial transmission potential of SARS-CoV infection was highlighted by a super-spreading event at the Prince of Wales Hospital (Shatin, Hong Kong), where 138 subjects (many of whom were previously healthy healthcare workers) contracted the disease within a 2-week period of exposure to a 26-year-old male (a visitor of the same hotel floor as the male renal physician), who was admitted to a general medical ward of the Prince of Wales Hospital on 4 March 2003 with fever and pneumonia [2, 53]. Multiple factors appeared to have contributed to this super-spreading event, including: the administration of nebulised salbutamol to the index patient *via* a jet nebuliser for its mucociliary clearance effects; an overcrowded ward environment; and inadequate air changes in the hospital ward [2, 53]. SARS-CoV was detected in the respiratory tract secretions, urine, faeces and tears of some patients with SARS-CoV infection [52, 54]. Furthermore, the temporal–spatial pattern of SARS-CoV infection spread among inpatients in the affected medical ward, supplemented by computational fluid dynamics (CFD) analysis, pointed to airborne transmission [55]. Environmental air samples taken from a hospital room in Toronto (ON, Canada) occupied by one patient with SARS-CoV infection, together with conventional surface swabs taken from a bed table and a television remote control in patients' rooms and a medication refrigerator door in a nurses', were found to be positive for SARS-CoV on PCR testing [56]. These data indicate the possibility of airborne transmission and emphasise the importance of appropriate respiratory protection in addition to strict surface hygiene practices.

A major community outbreak of SARS in Hong Kong, which involved >300 people, also appeared to have spread by opportunistic airborne transmission within a private residential complex, the Amoy Gardens (Kowloon, Hong Kong) [57, 58]. Drying of a "U-shaped" bathroom floor drain and backflow of contaminated sewage (from a SARS patient with renal failure and diarrhoea) related to negative pressure generated by the toilet exhaust fan might have created infectious aerosols that moved upward through the warm airshaft of the building. CFD modelling suggested possible dispersion by wind flow, causing long-range airborne transmission (>200 m) to nearby buildings [32].

In summary, SARS-CoV is predominantly spread through respiratory droplets but has the potential to transmit *via* an opportunistic airborne route through aerosol-generating procedures in healthcare facilities [52], and environmental factors as in the Amoy Gardens [57–59]. Other modes of transmission have been suggested, including faeco-oral (presence of virus in stool, and diarrhoea as a symptom) [57–59] and fomite on surfaces (virus found on surfaces in hospitals treating patients) [56]. The virus that spread worldwide was from a single strain [60].

Table 1 shows the timeline of the spread of SARS-CoV infection from China to Singapore, Vietnam and Canada *via* Hong Kong, with linkage to the hotel at which the Guangdong physician stayed [61].

Table 2 shows the global statistics of probable SARS-CoV infection.

Clinical manifestations

The estimated mean incubation period of SARS-CoV infection was 4.6 days (95% CI 3.8–5.8 days) [62], whereas 95% of illness onset was within 10 days [63]. The mean time from illness onset to hospitalisation was 2–8 days, and was shorter towards the later stages of the epidemic. The mean time from illness onset to the need for invasive mechanical ventilatory (IMV) support and death was 11 days and 23.7 days, respectively [62].

Many patients with SARS-CoV infection presented with persistent fever, myalgia, dry cough, chills/rigor, malaise, dyspnoea and headache. Sore throat, sputum production, rhinorrhea, nausea, vomiting and dizziness were much less frequent (table 3) [2, 5, 50, 64, 65]. Watery diarrhoea was present in 40–70% of SARS patients and tended to occur ~1 week after illness onset [28, 39].

Table 1. Timeline of spread of SARS-CoV infection from China to Canada, Vietnam and Singapore *via* Hong Kong

16 November 2002

First known case of atypical pneumonia in Foshan (Guangdong province, China). The aetiology was not identified until much later.

11 February 2003

The World Health Organization receives reports from the Chinese Ministry of Health of an outbreak of acute respiratory syndrome, with 300 cases and five deaths in Guangdong Province.

21 February 2003

A 64-year-old medical doctor from Zhongshan University in Guangzhou (Guangdong province) arrives in Hong Kong to attend a wedding.

22 February 2003

The Guangdong physician is admitted to the ICU of the Kwong Wah Hospital (Yau Ma Tei, Hong Kong) with respiratory failure (he had previously treated patients with atypical pneumonia in Guangdong). He warns medical staff that he might have contracted a "very virulent disease" with onset of symptoms on 15 February 2003.

26 February 2003

A 48-year-old Chinese–American businessman is admitted to the French Hospital in Hanoi (Vietnam) with a 3-day history of fever and respiratory symptoms. He travelled to Hong Kong on 17 February 2003, departed for Hanoi on 23 February 2003, and fell ill there. Shortly before his departure from Hong Kong, he had stayed on the same floor of the hotel as the Guangdong physician, in a room across the hall.

1 March 2003

A 26-year-old woman is admitted to a hospital in Singapore with respiratory symptoms. A resident of Singapore, she was a guest on the same floor of the hotel as the Guangdong physician, from 21 to 25 February 2003.

4 March 2003

The Guangdong doctor dies of atypical pneumonia at Kwong Wah Hospital.

5 March 2003

In Hanoi, the Chinese–American businessman, in a stable but critical condition, is air medivaced to the Princess Margaret Hospital (Kwai Chung, Hong Kong). Seven healthcare workers who had cared for him in Hanoi become ill.

A 78-year-old Toronto (ON, Canada) woman dies at Toronto's Scarborough Grace Hospital; on 23 February 2003, the woman had checked out of the hotel at which the Guangdong physician had stayed. Five members of her family were found to be infected and were admitted to the hospital.

7 March 2003

Healthcare workers at Hong Kong's Prince of Wales Hospital (Shatin, Hong Kong) start to complain of respiratory tract infection, progressing to pneumonia. All have an identifiable link to the same ward.

12 March 2003

The World Health Organization issues a global alert about cases of severe atypical pneumonia following mounting reports of spread among staff at hospitals in Hong Kong and Hanoi.

26 staff at the French Hospital in Hanoi report symptoms. Of these, 25 have either pneumonia or acute respiratory syndrome, and five are in a critical condition. The hospital is closed to new admissions.

Hong Kong health authorities formally report an outbreak of unidentified flu-like illness among hospital staff at the Prince of Wales Hospital. As of midnight 11 March 2003, 50 healthcare workers had been screened; 23 were found to have febrile illness and eight showed early chest radiography signs of pneumonia. A 26-year-old man, who had visited an acquaintance from 15 to 23 February 2003 who was staying on the same floor of the hotel as the Guangdong physician, is found to be the source of this hospital outbreak following subsequent epidemiological investigation.

13 March 2003

The Ministry of Health in Singapore reports three cases of atypical pneumonia in young women who had recently returned to Singapore after travelling to Hong Kong. All had stayed on the same floor of the hotel as the Guangdong physician in late February.

15 March 2003

The World Health Organization issues travel advice as evidence mounts that SARS is spreading by air travel along international routes. The World Health Organization names the mysterious illness after its symptoms, and declares it "a worldwide health threat."

Reproduced and modified from [61] with permission from the publisher.

Table 2. Summary of probable SARS cases with onset of illness from 1 November 2002 to 31 July 2003

Location	Female n	Male n	Total n	Age years	Deaths n#	Case fatality ratio	Imported cases n	HCW affected n	Onset date of first probable case	Onset date of last probable case
Australia	4	2	6	15 (1–45)	0	0%	6 (100%)	0 (0%)	26 February 2003	1 April 2003
Canada	151	100	251	49 (1–98)	43	17%	5 (2%)	109 (43%)	23 February 2003	12 June 2003
China	2674	2607	5327¶	Not available	349	7%	Not applicable	1002 (19%)	16 November 2002	3 June 2003
China, Hong Kong Special Administrative Region	977	778	1755	40 (0–100)	299	17%	Not applicable	386 (22%)	15 February 2003	31 May 2003
China, Macao Special Administrative Region	0	1	1	28	0	0%	1 (100%)	0 (0%)	5 May 2003	5 May 2003
China, Taiwan	218	128	346+	42 (0–93)	37	11%	21 (6%)	68 (20%)	25 February 2003	15 June 2003
France	1	6	7	49 (26–61)	1	14%	7 (100%)	2 (29%)§	21 March 2003	3 May 2003
Germany	4	5	9	44 (4–73)	0	0%	9 (100%)	1 (11%)	9 March 2003	6 May 2003
India	0	3	3	25 (25–30)	0	0%	3 (100%)	0 (0%)	25 April 2003	6 May 2003
Indonesia	0	2	2	56 (47–65)	0	0%	2 (100%)	0 (0%)	6 April 2003	17 April 2003
Italy	1	3	4	30.5 (25–54)	0	0%	4 (100%)	0 (0%)	12 March 2003	20 April 2003
Kuwait	1	0	1	50	0	0%	1 (100%)	0 (0%)	9 April 2003	9 April 2003
Malaysia	1	4	5	30 (26–84)	2	40%	5 (100%)	0 (0%)	14 March 2003	22 April 2003
Mongolia	8	1	9	32 (17–63)	0	0%	8 (89%)	0 (0%)	31 March 2003	6 May 2003
New Zealand	1	0	1	67	0	0%	1 (100%)	0 (0%)	20 April 2003	20 April 2003
Philippines	8	6	14	41 (29–73)	2	14%	7 (50%)	4 (29%)	25 February 2003	5 May 2003
Republic of Ireland	0	1	1	56	0	0%	1 (100%)	0 (0%)	27 February 2003	27 February 2003
Republic of Korea	0	3	3	40 (20–80)	0	0%	3 (100%)	0 (0%)	25 April 2003	10 May 2003
Romania	0	1	1	52	0	0%	1 (100%)	0 (0%)	19 March 2003	19 March 2003
Russian Federation	0	1	1	25	0	0%	Not available	0 (0%)	5 May 2003	5 May 2003
Singapore	161	77	238	35 (1–90)	33	14%	8 (3%)	97 (41%)	25 February 2003	5 May 2003
South Africa	0	1	1	62	1	100%	1 (100%)	0 (0%)	3 April 2003	3 April 2003
Spain	0	1	1	33	0	0%	1 (100%)	0 (0%)	26 March 2003	26 March 2003
Sweden	3	2	5	43 (33–55)	0	0%	5 (100%)	0 (0%)	28 March 2003	23 April 2003
Switzerland	0	1	1	35	0	0%	1 (100%)	0 (0%)	9 March 2003	9 March 2003
Thailand	5	4	9	42 (2–79)	2	22%	9 (100%)	1 (11%)§	11 March 2003	27 May 2003
UK	2	2	4	59 (28–74)	0	0%	4 (100%)	0 (0%)	1 March 2003	1 April 2003
USA	13	14	27	36 (0–83)	0	0%	27 (100%)	0 (0%)	24 February 2003	13 July 2003f
Vietnam	39	24	63	43 (20–76)	5	8%	1 (2%)	36 (57%)	23 February 2003	14 April 2003
Total			8096		774	9.6%	142	1706		

Data are presented as median (range), unless otherwise stated. HCW: healthcare worker. #: only includes cases whose death was attributed to SARS. ¶: case classification by sex was unknown for 46 cases. +: since 11 July 2003, 325 cases have been discarded in Taiwan, China. Laboratory information was insufficient or incomplete for 135 discarded cases, of which 101 died. §: includes HCWs who acquired illness in other areas. f: due to differences in case definitions, the USA has reported probable cases of SARS with onset of illness after 5 July 2003. Reproduced and modified from [1] with permission from the publisher.

SARS-CoV was detected in the serum and cerebrospinal fluid of two patients complicated with status epilepticus [66, 67] Older patients with SARS-CoV infection presented with poor appetite, a decrease in general well-being, a fall, a fracture [68] and confusion, whereas high fever was sometimes absent. In contrast, illness in children aged <12 years was milder, although teenagers sometimes developed systemic symptoms, such as myalgia, chills, rigours, headache and dyspnoea, resembling those of adults [69]. Young children and teenagers all survived [69, 70], but there was a case fatality rate of 25% for SARS-CoV infection during pregnancy, which was associated with high incidence of spontaneous abortion, preterm delivery, and intrauterine growth retardation without perinatal SARS-CoV infection among newborn infants [71]. Asymptomatic SARS-CoV infection was uncommon, as a meta-analysis had shown overall sero-prevalence rates of 0.1% (95% CI 0.02–0.18) for the general population and 0.23% (95% CI 0.02–0.45) for healthcare workers (HCWs), compared with healthy blood donors, others from the general community or patients without SARS-CoV infection recruited from the healthcare setting (0.16% (95% CI 0–0.37)) [72].

The clinical course of patients with SARS-CoV infection appeared to manifest in different stages [2, 39, 51, 73]. In the first week of illness, many patients presented with fever, dry cough, myalgia and malaise, all of which might improve despite the presence of lung consolidation and rising viral loads on serial samples. During the second week, many patients experienced recurrence of fever, worsening consolidation and respiratory failure, while ~20% progressed to ARDS requiring IMV support [2, 39]. Viral load peaked on day 10 of illness, which was found to correspond temporally with a peak in the extent of consolidation radiographically [74], and a maximal risk of nosocomial transmission, particularly to HCWs [75].

Diagnosis and investigations

Laboratory diagnosis

Diagnosis of SARS-CoV infecton is principally by PCR on samples from patients with suspected disease. The detection rates for SARS-CoV infection using RT-PCR in nasopharyngeal

Table 3. Clinical features of SARS on presentation

Symptom	Patients with symptom
Persistent fever >38°C	99–100%
Non-productive cough	57–75%
Myalgia	45–61%
Chills/rigor	15–73%
Headache	20–56%
Dyspnoea	40–42%
Malaise	31–45%
Nausea and vomiting	20–35%
Diarrhoea	20–25%
Sore throat	13–25%
Dizziness	4.2–43%
Sputum production	4.9–29%
Rhinorrhoea	2.1–23%
Arthralgia	10.4%

Data from [1–3, 5, 6, 39, 50, 52, 62].

specimens, urine, stool and blood are shown in table 4 [39, 76–79]. It is recommended that a combination of upper respiratory (nasal, pharyngeal, nasopharyngeal), lower respiratory (higher yield because of higher viral levels, *e.g.* sputum, tracheal aspirate, bronchoalveolar lavage), blood and fecal specimens should be collected to maximise the chance of detection. A single negative test in an upper respiratory specimen would be insufficient to rule out the diagnosis. As viral kinetics demonstrated an inverted V-shaped curve that peaked on day 10 of illness with a progressive decrease in rates of viral shedding from the nasopharynx, stool and urine (which might persist up to day 21), clinical progression during the second week was believed to be at least partially caused by immune-mediated lung injury [39].

Viral culture may provide further confirmation but it is too slow to assist clinical management and needs to be performed in facilities at biosafety level 3. Serological diagnosis is largely retrospective but may be useful for epidemiological surveillance purposes. Higher IgG levels were detected in patients who required supplemental oxygen, patients who were admitted to ICU, patients with negative pre-discharge fecal RT-PCR results, and those with lymphopenia at presentation; this indicated a more robust IgG response in severe infections [80]. A study in Beijing (China) showed that 6 years post-infection, SARS-specific IgG Ab eventually vanished and peripheral memory B-cell responses became undetectable in recovered SARS patients; in contrast, specific T-cell anamnestic responses could be maintained for $\geqslant$6 years [81].

Several abnormal laboratory parameters were frequently observed in patients with SARS-CoV infection, including lymphopenia, low-grade disseminated intravascular coagulation, elevated lactate dehydrogenase (LDH), alanine transaminases (ALT) and creatinine phosphokinase [2, 3, 5, 39, 50]. Absolute lymphopenia (lymphocyte count $<1.0\times10^{9}\cdot L^{-1}$) was observed in 98% of cases of SARS-CoV infection, whereas low CD4 and CD8 lymphocyte counts on hospitalisation were associated with unfavourable clinical outcomes [82]. Liver dysfunction with abnormal ALT was noted in 29.6% of patients on presentation but increased to 75.9% of those receiving systemic corticosteroid and ribavirin for treatment of SARS-CoV infection [83].

Radiological features

The radiographic features of SARS-CoV infection were nonspecific. About a quarter of patients might have no apparent abnormality on their initial chest radiographs [2, 5, 50, 84], whereas high-resolution computed tomography (HRCT) of the thorax would help

Table 4. Diagnostic tests for SARS-CoV

RT-PCR	Detection rate
Nasopharyngeal aspirate	
Conventional RT-PCR [39]	32% day 3, 68% day 14
Second-generation with real-time quantitative RT-PCR assay [76]	80% during first 3 days
Stool [39]	97% day 14
Urine [39]	42% day 15
Real-time quantitative serum SARS-CoV RNA [77–79]	80% day 1, 75% day 7, 45% day 14
Serology IgG seroconversion to SARS-CoV [39]	15% day 15, 60% day 21, >90% day 28

detect small parenchymal opacities early [85]. Common HRCT findings included interlobular septal and intra-lobular interstitial thickening, consolidation and ground-glass opacification, predominantly involving the lung periphery and lower lobes, which closely resembled that found in COP or BOOP [2, 85]. Lung cyst formation has been observed in severe ARDS induced by SARS-CoV infection [86].

The initial extent of opacification on chest radiograph increased by about one lung zone every 4–5 days during the first 11 days of illness. This might have some prognostic value because radiographic progression correlated well with changes of important clinical and laboratory parameters (such as LDH level, the ratio of arterial oxygen tension to the fraction of inspired oxygen, lymphocyte count, and neutrophil count) at each time point and in terms of changes between time points [84]. In a case series of critically ill patients, 12% of ICU cases developed pneumo-mediastinum spontaneously, whereas 20% developed evidence of ARDS over a period of 3 weeks [39]. Despite the use of lung protective IMV with low tidal volume, barotrauma occurred in 26% of critically ill SARS-CoV cases, possibly due to decreased lung compliance [87].

Prognostic markers and outcome

The prognostic factors associated with a poor outcome (ICU admission or death) in SARS-CoV infection are listed in table 5 [2, 5, 39, 63–65, 76–79, 88, 89]. Infants (preterm or full-term) born to mothers with SARS-CoV infection neither shed SARS-CoV nor were clinically infected in the post-natal period [88]. However, the clinical course of SARS-CoV infection in elderly patients, particularly those with underlying conditions, was typically fulminant and often fatal. The overall death rate of SARS-CoV infection was 6–16%. However, the age-stratified case fatality rates were as follows: <25 years of age, <1%; 25–44 years, 6%; 45–64 years, 15%; and ⩾65 years, >50% [89].

Antiviral therapy and other potential treatments

Antiviral therapy

Two groups of pharmacological agents were used empirically for the treatment of SARS during the 2003 outbreak, including antiviral agents and immune modulators. Antiviral

Table 5. Poor prognostic factors associated with ICU admission and/or deaths in patients with SARS-CoV infection

Advanced age [2, 39, 63–65]
Viral loads
- High viral loads in nasopharyngeal secretions [39]
- High plasma SARS-CoV concentrations [77–79]

Comorbidities
- Chronic hepatitis B [39]
- Diabetes mellitus or other comorbid conditions [5, 64]

Laboratory markers
- High peak lactate dehydrogenase [2]
- High initial lactate dehydrogenase level [65]
- High neutrophil count on presentation [2, 65]
- Low counts of CD4 and CD8 at presentation [82]

agents that were used to treat SARS-CoV infection, including ribavirin, protease inhibitors and IFN, are summarised in table 6 [5, 89, 91, 96–98]. However, due to a lack of prospective randomised, placebo-controlled clinical trial data, none of these therapies have a proven benefit. Good supportive care remains the mainstay of treatment for SARS-CoV infection.

Ribavirin

Ribavirin is a nucleoside analogue that was widely prescribed for treatment of SARS-CoV infection in 2003 [2, 5, 6, 39, 64, 99]. Nevertheless, ribavirin alone had minimal activity against SARS-CoV with concentrations that could be achieved in the clinical setting, and it led to significant haemolysis in many patients [2, 5, 89]. Agents with antiviral effects *in vitro* and in animals are shown in table 6 [26, 38, 90–98].

Systemic corticosteroids: the controversy

Intravenous pulse methylprednisolone (MP) was given to numerous patients with SARS-CoV infection, with the aim of reducing immuno-pathological lung injury [2, 39, 64, 65, 89, 100], based on the assumption that clinical progression of pneumonia and respiratory failure in association with peak SARS-CoV viral load might be mediated by the host inflammatory response [39, 74]. Furthermore, there were HRCT features of BOOP [2, 50, 85], which were also noted histologically in some patients [37]. Systemic corticosteroids significantly reduced IL-8, MCP-1 and IP-10 concentrations from 5 to 8 days after treatment in 20 adults with SARS-CoV infection [41]. In addition, in patients with fatal SARS-CoV infection, there was evidence of haemo-phagocytosis in the lungs [35], attributed to cytokine dysregulation [101]. Intervention with systemic corticosteroids was given with the aim of modulating these immune responses [102].

Although there appeared to be clinical improvement in some patients, with resolution of fever and lung consolidation following treatment with intravenous pulsed MP [2, 89], a retrospective cohort analysis showed that the use of pulsed MP was actually associated with an increased risk of 30-day mortality (adjusted OR 26.0 (95% CI 4.4–154.8)) [103]. In addition, prolonged systemic corticosteroid therapy could increase the risk of developing nosocomial infections, such as disseminated fungal disease [104], metabolic derangements, psychosis and even avascular necrosis of bones [105]. An RCT showed that plasma SARS-CoV RNA concentrations in the second and third weeks of illness were higher in patients given initial hydrocortisone (n=10) than those given normal saline as control (n=7) during the early clinical course of illness [106]. Despite the small sample size of the study, the data suggest that systemic corticosteroids given early in the course of SARS-CoV infection might prolong viraemia [106]. A systematic review concluded that corticosteroid treatment was not associated with definite benefits and was potentially harmful [107]. All these data call for caution when managing patients with severe acute viral respiratory infections such as SARS, MERS and influenza [108, 109].

Convalescent plasma/passive immunotherapy

Convalescent plasma, donated by patients who had fully recovered from SARS-CoV infection, appeared clinically useful for treating other patients with progressive SARS-CoV infection [110, 111]. In a study that compared SARS-CoV patients who did and did not receive convalescent plasma, 19 patients who received such therapy had better survival

Table 6. Agents with activity against SARS-CoV

Agents with *in vitro* and animal data	Agents with human data
Glycyrrhizin This active component of liquorice roots actively inhibited SARS-CoV *in vitro* but there has been no *in vivo* data [90].	**Ribavirin** After 2 weeks of ribavirin treatment (1.2 g three times a day orally), 59% of patients experienced a fall in haemoglobin of >2 g·dL^{-1} from baseline; evidence of haemolysis was documented in 36% [89]. The use of ribavirin for SARS in Toronto (ON, Canada), based on a higher dosage for treating haemorrhagic fever virus, was associated with even more toxicity, including elevated transaminases and bradycardia [5].
Protease inhibitor *In vitro* activity against SARS-CoV was noted for lopinavir and ribavirin at 4 µg·mL^{-1} and 50 µg·mL^{-1}, respectively, after 48 h of incubation. Cytopathic inhibition was achieved down to a concentration of lopinavir of 1 µg·mL^{-1} combined with 6.25 µg·mL^{-1} of ribavirin, suggesting that this combination might be synergistic against SARS-CoV *in vivo* [91].	**Protease inhibitor** Two retrospective, matched cohort studies compared the clinical outcome of patients who received protease inhibitor (lopinavir 400 mg, ritonavir 100 mg) in addition to ribavirin, either as initial therapy within 5 days of onset of symptoms or as rescue therapy after pulse methylprednisolone treatment for worsening respiratory symptoms. These were compared with historical controls who received ribavirin alone as initial antiviral therapy [91, 96]. The addition of lopinavir/ritonavir as initial therapy was associated with a reduction both in the overall death rate (2.3%) and the intubation rate (0%), when compared with a matched cohort that received standard treatment (15.6% and 11%, respectively) [96]. There was also evidence of a reduction in viral loads. Other beneficial effects included a reduction in methylprednisolone use and fewer nosocomial infections [91]. However, the subgroup that had received lopinavir/ritonavir as rescue therapy was no better than the matched cohort, and received a higher mean dose of methylprednisolone [96]. The improved clinical outcome in patients who received lopinavir/ritonavir as part of the initial therapy was supported by the observations that both peak (9.6 µg·mL^{-1}) and trough (5.5 µg·mL^{-1}) serum concentrations of lopinavir could inhibit the virus [97].

Continued

Table 6. Continued

Agents with *in vitro* and animal data	Agents with human data
IFN Type I IFNs such as IFN-α were produced early as part of the innate immune response to virus infections. Type I IFNs inhibited a wide range of RNA and DNA viruses, including SARS-CoV *in vitro* [92–94]. Complete inhibition of cytopathic effects of SARS-CoV in culture was observed for IFN subtypes β-1b, α-n1 and α-n3, and human leukocyte IFN-α [93]. IFN-α showed an *in vitro* inhibitory effect on SARS-CoV, starting at concentrations of 1000 $IU \cdot mL^{-1}$ [92]. In experimentally infected cynomolgus macaques with SARS-CoV, prophylactic treatment with pegylated IFN-α significantly reduced viral replication and excretion, viral antigen expression by type 1 pneumocytes and pulmonary damage, compared with untreated macaques, whereas post-exposure treatment with pegylated IFN-α yielded intermediate results [38].	**IFN** In a study in Toronto (ON, Canada), IFN-alfacon-1 given within 5 days of illness resulted in improved oxygen saturation, more rapid resolution of radiographic lung opacities and lower rates of intubation (11.1% *versus* 23.1%) and death (0.0% *versus* 7.7%); however, the study was small (nine *versus* 13 patients on systemic corticosteroid alone as controls) and confounded by the use of systemic corticosteroid [98].
Human monoclonal antibody against SARS-CoV S1 protein Since SARS-CoV infection was initiated through binding of S1 protein to the ACE2 receptor [26], a high-affinity HuMab has been identified against the SARS-CoV S1 protein termed 80R, which has potent neutralising activity *in vitro* and *in vivo* [95]. HuMab 80R was shown to efficiently neutralise SARS-CoV and inhibit syncytia formation between cells expressing the S protein and those expressing the SARS-CoV receptor ACE2. HuMab 80R may be a useful viral entry inhibitor for the emergency prophylaxis and treatment of SARS [95].	

ACE: angiotensin-converting enzyme; HuMab: human monoclonal antibody.

(100% *versus* 66.2%) and discharge (77.8% *versus* 23.0%) rates compared with 21 controls [111]. An exploratory *post-hoc* meta-analysis of studies of SARS-CoV infection and severe influenza showed a significant reduction in the pooled odds of mortality following convalescent plasma *versus* placebo or no treatment (OR 0.25 (95% CI 0.14–0.45)) [112]. Early administration of convalescent plasma is important; in 80 patients with SARS-CoV infection who were given convalescent plasma at the Prince of Wales Hospital, the discharge rate at day 22 was 58.3% for patients (n=48) treated within 14 days of illness onset *versus* 15.6% for those (n=32) treated beyond 14 days [110]. In a study comparing the immunogenicity and protection efficacy of recombinant proteins corresponding to different domains of the SARS-CoV S protein, all the mice vaccinated with S1, S1-foldon, S,or S-foldon were completely protected [113]. In the absence of well-proven and effective antiviral therapy, convalescent plasma and human monoclonal antibodies [112, 114] are worth further study against SARS-CoV if it returns.

End-points for monitoring therapy

Based on clinical experience of SARS-CoV infection management, treatment end-points should aim to achieve defervescence, resolution of lung consolidation and oxygen independence [89]. Serial chest radiographs should be monitored regularly beyond clinical observations [84]. As several blood markers such as LDH [2, 65] and lymphocyte subsets [82] were reported to have prognostic implications, these might be useful parameters to monitor progress. Apart from age, serum LD1 isoenzyme appeared to be the best prognostic indicator for predicting death in patients with SARS compared with serum total LDH activity and blood counts [115]. In addition, quantification of SARS-CoV RNA levels in serum and respiratory secretion represents a useful tool for prognostic purposes, whereas viral load decline and clearance should be monitored [78, 79].

Vaccines

Different vaccines, such as whole killed vaccine, adenovirus vector vaccine and recombinant spike protein vaccine, have been tested. The S protein of SARS-CoV plays a central role in mediating viral infection *via* receptor binding and membrane fusion between the virion and the host cell, and is a major epitope. An adenoviral-based vaccine could induce strong SARS-CoV specific immune responses in rhesus macaques, and holds promise for the development of a protective vaccine against SARS-CoV [116]. Other research groups reported that the S gene DNA vaccine could induce the production of specific IgG antibody against SARS-CoV efficiently in mice with a seroconversion ratio of 75% after three doses of immunisation [117]. Viral replication was reduced by more than 6 orders of magnitude in the lungs of mice vaccinated with S plasmid DNA expression vectors, and protection was mediated by a humoral immune mechanism [118]. Recombinant S protein exhibited antigenicity and receptor-binding ability [119], whereas synthetic peptides eliciting specific antibodies against SARS-CoV S protein might provide another approach for further developing SARS vaccine [120].

Prevention

General preventive measures

As there is no effective antiviral treatment and vaccine available, prevention of transmission is an important measure in the management of this highly infectious disease. As the primary mode of transmission of SARS-CoV infection is through direct contact and exposure to infectious respiratory droplets, or fomites, it is important to maintain good personal and environmental hygiene, and implement strict contact and droplet precautions among HCWs. Public education, contact tracing and quarantine/isolation of close contacts are important measures in the prevention of community transmission [52]. Following the detection of four new cases of SARS-CoV infection between 16 December 2003 and 30 January 2004 with linkage between humans and small wild animals [23, 48], the Guangdong government and Department of Public Health took public health measures, applying strict control to the wildlife market, including a ban on the rearing, sale, transport, slaughter and food processing of small wild mammals and civet cats [121].

Hospital infection control measures

Nosocomial infection of SARS involving HCWs was common in 2003, as shown by the fact that 1706 (21%) of 8096 SARS patients were HCWs [1]. A likely explanation is that viral loads increased to peak levels on day 10 after disease onset when the patient was most symptomatic and dyspnoeic, and required close attention by HCWs in hospital [39]. It is important to designate separate wards for patient triage (for undifferentiated fever), confirmed SARS cases and patients in whom SARS has been ruled out [122]. If a nosocomial outbreak is detected late, it is suggested that a hospital may need to be closed in order to contain spread of the disease, whereas outbreaks detected early and involving few patients may be managed by either removing all exposed persons to a designated location or isolating them in place [123]. Early case detection and isolation should be performed in negative pressure room facilities if available, and strict airborne precautions (good hand hygiene and wearing a gown, gloves, an N95 mask and eye protection) among HCWs are important, particularly when patients are seriously ill (*e.g.* receiving high-flow oxygen therapy) and when aerosol-generating procedures are applied [124].

The practice of droplet and contact precaution seemed adequate in reducing the risk of infection after general exposure to patients with mild SARS [125]. Significant independent risk factors for SARS infection were: perceived inadequacy of personal protective equipment; <2 h infection control training; and inconsistent use of personal protective equipment when in contact with SARS patients [126]. A case–control study involving 124 medical wards in 26 hospitals in Hong Kong and Guangzhou identified independent factors of super-spreading nosocomial outbreaks of SARS (table 7): the performance of resuscitation; a minimum

Table 7. Independent risk factors of super-spreading nosocomial outbreaks of SARS

Risk factors	OR (95% CI)	p-value
Performance of resuscitation	3.81 (1.04–13.87)	0.04
Staff working while experiencing symptoms	10.55 (2.28–48.87)	0.003
SARS patients requiring oxygen therapy	4.30 (1.00–18.43)	0.05
SARS patients requiring noninvasive positive pressure ventilation	11.82 (1.97–70.80)	0.007
Minimum distance between beds <1 m	6.94 (1.68–28.75)	0.008
Washing or changing facilities for staff	0.12 (0.02–0.97)	0.05

Reproduced and modified from [127] with permission from the publisher.

distance between beds of <1 m; staff working while experience symptoms; SARS patients requiring oxygen therapy; SARS patients requiring noninvasive ventilation. The availability of washing or changing facilities for staff was a protective factor [127]. A systematic review has shown that four aerosol-generating procedures increase the risk of nosocomial SARS transmission to HCWs: tracheal intubation; noninvasive ventilation; tracheotomy; and manual ventilation before intubation [128]. If these aerosol-generating procedures are to be performed, then airborne precaution is needed.

Conclusion

The major outbreak of SARS in 2003 resulted in an adverse impact on health systems, business, tourism and the global economy. Although no major outbreak or secondary spread occurred (despite the re-emergence of SARS amongst laboratory personnel in Singapore [129] and Taiwan [130], and in four residents in Guangdong [23, 48]), an epidemic is possible if there is any breach of laboratory biosafety guidelines, in the event of bioterrorism or with the possible emergence/mutation of other SARS-like clusters of circulating CoVs in bat populations [131]. Currently, the appropriate treatment for different clinical stages of SARS remains uncertain. RCTs of different treatment modalities must be put in place in preparation for a return of this highly infectious disease and the emergence of other SARS-like CoV.

References

1. WHO. Summary of probable SARS cases with onset of illness from 1 November to 31 July 2003. www.who.int/csr/sars/country/table2004_04_21/en/. Date last accessed: January 10, 2016. Date last updated: December 31, 2003.
2. Lee N, Hui DS, Wu A, *et al.* A major outbreak of severe acute respiratory syndrome in Hong Kong. *N Engl J Med* 2003; 348: 1986–1994.
3. Twu SJ, Chen TJ, Chen CJ, *et al.* Control measures for severe acute respiratory syndrome (SARS) in Taiwan. *Emerg Infect Dis* 2003; 9: 718–720.
4. Reilley B, Van Herp M, Sermand D, *et al.* SARS and Carlo Urbani. *N Engl J Med* 2003; 348: 1951–1952.
5. Booth CM, Matukas LM, Tomlinson GA, *et al.* Clinical features and short-term outcomes of 144 patients with SARS in the greater Toronto area. *JAMA* 2003; 289: 2801–2809.
6. Hsu LY, Lee CC, Green JA, *et al.* Severe acute respiratory syndrome in Singapore: clinical features of index patient and initial contacts. *Emerg Infect Dis* 2003; 9: 713–717.
7. CDC Update. Severe acute respiratory syndrome – worldwide and United States 2003. *MMWR Wkly* 2003; 52: 664–665.
8. SARS: lessons from a new disease. *In*: The World Health Report 2003: Shaping the Future. Switzerland, World Health Organization, 2003; pp. 71–78.
9. Zumla A, Chan JF, Azhar EI, *et al.* Coronaviruses – drug discovery and therapeutic options. *Nat Rev Drug Discov* 2016; in press [DOI: 10.1038/nrd.2015.37].
10. Drosten C, Gunther S, Preiser W, *et al.* Identification of a novel coronavirus in patients with severe acute respiratory syndrome. *N Engl J Med* 2003; 348: 1967–1976.
11. Ksiazek TG, Erdman D, Goldsmith CS, *et al.* A novel coronavirus associated with severe acute respiratory syndrome. *N Engl J Med* 2003; 348: 1953–1966.
12. Kuiken T, Fouchier RA, Schutten M, *et al.* Newly discovered coronavirus as the primary cause of severe acute respiratory syndrome. *Lancet* 2003; 362: 263–270.
13. Rota PA, Oberste MS, Monroe SS, *et al.* Characterization of a novel coronavirus associated with severe acute respiratory syndrome. *Science* 2003; 300: 1394–1399.
14. Marra MA, Jones SJ, Astell CR, *et al.* The genome sequence of the SARS-associated coronavirus. *Science* 2003; 300: 1399–1404.
15. Ruan YJ, Wei CL, Ee LA, *et al.* Comparative full-length genome sequence analysis of 14 SARS coronavirus isolates and common mutations associated with putative origins of infection. *Lancet* 2003; 361: 1779–1785.
16. Du L, Qiu JC, Wang M, *et al.* Analysis on the characteristics of blood serum Ab-IgG detective result of severe acute respiratory syndrome patients in Guangzhou, China. *Zhonghua Liu Xing Bing Xue Za Zhi* 2004; 25: 925–928.

17. Guan Y, Zheng BJ, He YQ, *et al.* Isolation and characterization of viruses related to the SARS coronavirus from animals in southern China. *Science* 2003; 302: 276–278.
18. Yu D, Li H, Xu R, *et al.* CDC. Prevalence of IgG antibody to SARS-associated coronavirus in animal traders – Guangdong province, China, 2003. *Morb Mortal Wkly Rep* 2003; 52: 986–987.
19. Song HD, Tu CC, Zhang GW, *et al.* Cross-host evolution of severe acute respiratory syndrome coronavirus in palm civet and human. *Proc Natl Acad Sci USA* 2005; 102: 2430–2435.
20. Wang M, Yan M, Xu H, *et al.* SARS-CoV infection in a restaurant from palm civet. *Emerg Infect Dis* 2005; 11: 1860–1865.
21. Lau SK, Woo PC, Li KS, *et al.* Severe acute respiratory syndrome coronavirus-like virus in Chinese horseshoe bats. *Proc Natl Acad Sci USA* 2005; 102: 14040–14045.
22. Li W, Shi Z, Yu M, *et al.* Bats are natural reservoirs of SARS-like coronaviruses. *Science* 2005; 310: 676–679.
23. Shi Z, Hu Z. A review of studies on animal reservoirs of the SARS coronavirus. *Virus Res* 2008; 133: 74–87.
24. Chan PK, To KF, Lo AW, *et al.* Persistent infection of SARS coronavirus in colonic cells *in vitro*. *J Med Virol* 2004; 74: 1–7.
25. Simmons G, Gosalia DN, Rennekamp AJ, *et al.* Inhibitors of cathepsin L prevent severe acute respiratory syndrome coronavirus entry. *Proc Natl Acad Sci USA* 2005; 102: 11876–11881.
26. Li W, Moore MJ, Vasilieva N, *et al.* Angiotensin-converting enzyme 2 is a functional receptor for the SARS coronavirus. *Nature* 2003; 426: 450–454.
27. Hamming I, Timens W, Bulthuis ML, *et al.* Tissue distribution of ACE2 protein, the functional receptor for SARS coronavirus. A first step in understanding SARS pathogenesis. *J Pathol* 2004; 203: 631–637.
28. Leung WK, To KF, Chan PK, *et al.* Enteric involvement of severe acute respiratory syndrome-associated coronavirus infection. Gastroenterology 2003; 125: 1011–1017.
29. Chan VS, Chan KY, Chen Y, *et al.* Homozygous L-SIGN (CLEC4M) plays a protective role in SARS coronavirus infection. *Nat Genet* 2006; 38: 38–46.
30. Tang NL, Chan PK, Hui DS, *et al.* Lack of support for an association between CLEC4M homozygosity and protection against SARS coronavirus infection. *Nat Genet* 2007; 39: 691–692.
31. Zhi L, Zhou G, Zhang H, *et al.* Lack of support for an association between CLEC4M homozygosity and protection against SARS coronavirus infection. *Nat Genet* 2007; 39: 692–694.
32. Kuba K, Imai Y, Rao S, *et al.* A crucial role of angiotensin converting enzyme 2 (ACE2) in SARS coronavirus-induced lung injury. *Nat Med* 2005; 11: 875–879.
33. Law PT, Wong CH, Au TC, *et al.* The 3a protein of severe acute respiratory syndrome-associated coronavirus induces apoptosis in Vero E6 cells. *J Gen Virol* 2005; 86: 1921–1930.
34. Tan YJ, Fielding BC, Goh PY, *et al.* Overexpression of 7a, a protein specifically encoded by the severe acute respiratory syndrome coronavirus, induces apoptosis *via* a caspase-dependent pathway. *J Virol* 2004; 78: 14043–14047.
35. Nicholls JM, Poon LL, Lee KC, *et al.* Lung pathology of fatal severe acute respiratory syndrome. *Lancet* 2003; 361: 1773–1778.
36. Franks TJ, Chong PY, Chui P, *et al.* Lung pathology of severe acute respiratory syndrome (SARS): a study of 8 autopsy cases from Singapore. *Hum Pathol* 2003; 34: 743–748.
37. Tse GM, To KF, Chan PK, *et al.* Pulmonary pathological features in coronavirus associated severe acute respiratory syndrome (SARS). *J Clin Pathol* 2004; 57: 260–265.
38. Haagmans BL, Kuiken T, Martina BE, *et al.* Pegulated interferon-a protects type I pneumocytes against SARS coronavirus infection in macaques. *Nature Med* 2004; 10: 290–293.
39. Peiris JS, Chu CM, Cheng VC, *et al.* Clinical progression and viral load in a community outbreak of coronavirus-associated SARS pneumonia: a prospective study. *Lancet* 2003; 361: 1767–1772.
40. Cheng VC, Hung IF, Tang BS, *et al.* Viral replication in the nasopharynx is associated with diarrhea in patients with severe acute respiratory syndrome. *Clin Inf Dis* 2004; 38: 467–475.
41. Wong CK, Lam CWK, Wu AK, *et al.* Plasma inflammatory cytokines and chemokines in severe acute respiratory syndrome. *Clin Exp Immunol* 2004; 136: 95–103.
42. Zhao J, Zhao J, Perlman S. T cell responses are required for protection from clinical disease and for virus clearance in severe acute respiratory syndrome coronavirus-infected mice. *J Virol* 2010; 84: 9318–9325.
43. Channappanavar R, Fehr AR, Vijay R, *et al.* Dysregulated type I interferon and inflammatory monocyte-macrophage responses cause lethal pneumonia in SARS-CoV-infected mice. *Cell Host Microbe* 2016; 19: 181–193.
44. Totura AL, Whitmore A, Agnihothram S, *et al.* Toll-Like receptor 3 signaling *via* TRIF contributes to a protective innate immune response to severe acute respiratory syndrome coronavirus infection. *MBio* 2015; 6: e00638–15.
45. Wang Y, Liu L. The membrane protein of severe acute respiratory syndrome coronavirus functions as a novel cytosolic pathogen-associated molecular pattern to promote beta interferon induction *via* a toll-like-receptor-related TRAF3-independent mechanism. *MBio* 2016; 7. pii: e01872-15.
46. Tang F, Liu W, Zhang F, *et al.* IL-12 RB1 genetic variants contribute to human susceptibility to severe acute respiratory syndrome infection among Chinese. *PLoS One* 2008; 3: e2183.

47. Ip WK, Chan KH, Law HK, *et al.* Mannose-binding lectin in severe acute respiratory syndrome coronavirus infection. *J Infect Dis* 2005; 191: 1697–1704.
48. Zhao Z, Zhang F, Xu M, *et al.* Description and clinical treatment of an early outbreak of severe acute respiratory syndrome (SARS) in Guangzhou, PR China. *J Med Microbiol* 2003; 52: 715–720.
49. Zhong NS, Zheng BJ, Li YM, *et al.* Epidemiology and cause of severe acute respiratory syndrome in Guangdong, People's Republic of China, in Feb 2003. *Lancet* 2003; 362: 1353–1358.
50. Tsang KW, Ho PL, Ooi GC, *et al.* A cluster of cases of severe acute respiratory syndrome in Hong Kong. *N Engl J Med* 2003; 348: 1977–1985.
51. Hui DS, Sung JJ. Severe acute respiratory syndrome. *Chest* 2003; 124: 12–15.
52. Peiris JS, Yuen KY, Osterhaus AD, *et al.* The severe acute respiratory syndrome. *N Engl J Med* 2003; 349: 2431–2441.
53. Wong RS, Hui DS. Index patient and SARS outbreak in Hong Kong. *Emerg Infect Dis* 2004; 10: 339–341.
54. Loon SC, Teoh SC, Oon LL, *et al.* The severe acute respiratory syndrome coronavirus in tears. *Br J Ophthalmol* 2004; 88: 861–863.
55. Yu IT, Wong TW, Chiu YL, *et al.* Temporal-spatial analysis of severe acute respiratory syndrome among hospital inpatients. *Clin Infect Dis* 2005; 40: 1237–1243.
56. Booth TF, Kournikakis B, Bastien N, *et al.* Detection of airborne severe acute respiratory syndrome (SARS) coronavirus and environmental contamination in SARS outbreak units. *J Infect Dis* 2005; 191: 1472–1477.
57. Chu CM, Cheng VC, Hung IF, *et al.* Viral load distribution in SARS outbreak. *Emerg Infect Dis* 2005; 11: 1882–1886.
58. Yu IT, Li Y, Wong TW, *et al.* Evidence of airborne transmission of the severe acute respiratory syndrome virus. *N Engl J Med* 2004; 350: 1731–1739.
59. Yu IT, Qiu H, Tse LA, *et al.* Severe acute respiratory syndrome beyond Amoy Gardens: completing the incomplete legacy. *Clin Infect Dis* 2014; 58: 683–686.
60. Lloyd-Smith JO, Schreiber SJ, Kopp PE, *et al.* Superspreading and the effect of individual variation on disease emergence. *Nature* 2005; 438: 355–359.
61. WHO. Update 95-SARS: chronology of a serial killer. www.who.int/csr/don/2003_07_04/en. Date last accessed: January 10, 2016.
62. Leung GM, Hedley AJ, Ho LM, *et al.* The epidemiology of severe acute respiratory syndrome in the 2003 Hong Kong epidemic: an analysis of all 1755 patients. *Ann Intern Med* 2004; 141: 662–673.
63. Donnelly CA, Ghani AV, Leung GM, *et al.* Epidemiological determinants of spread of causal agent of severe acute respiratory syndrome in Hong Kong. *Lancet* 2003; 361: 1761–1766.
64. Chan JW, Ng CK, Chan YH, *et al.* Short term outcome and risk factors for adverse clinical outcomes in adults with severe acute respiratory syndrome (SARS). *Thorax* 2003; 58: 686–689.
65. Tsui PT, Kwok ML, Yuen H, *et al.* Severe acute respiratory syndrome: clinical outcome and prognostic correlates. *Emerg infect Dis* 2003; 9: 1064–1069.
66. Hung EC, Chim SS, Chan PK, *et al.* Detection of SARS coronavirus RNA in the cerebrospinal fluid of a patient with severe acute respiratory syndrome. *Clin Chem* 2003; 49: 2108–2109.
67. Lau KK, Yu WC, Chu CM, *et al.* Possible central nervous system infection by SARS coronavirus. *Emerg Infect Dis* 2004; 10: 342–344.
68. Wong KC, Leung KS, Hui M. Severe acute respiratory syndrome (SARS) in a geriatric patient with a hip fracture. A case report. *J Bone Joint Surg Am* 2003; 85A: 1339–1342.
69. Hon KL, Leung CW, Cheng WT, *et al.* Clinical presentations and outcome of severe acute respiratory syndrome in children. *Lancet* 2003; 561: 1701–1703.
70. Chiu WK, Cheung PCH, Ng KL, *et al.* Severe acute respiratory syndrome in children: experience in a regional hospital in Hong Kong. *Pediatr Crit Care Med* 2003; 4: 279–283.
71. Wong SF, Chow KM, Leung TN, *et al.* Pregnancy and perinatal outcomes of women with severe acute respiratory syndrome. *Am J Obstet Gynecol* 2004; 191: 292–297.
72. Leung GM, Lim WW, Ho LM, *et al.* Seroprevalence of IgG antibodies to SARS-coronavirus in asymptomatic or subclinical population groups. *Epidemiol Infect* 2006; 134: 211–221.
73. Hui DS, Wong PC, Wang C. SARS: clinical features and diagnosis. *Respirology* 2003; 8: Suppl., S20–S24.
74. Hui DS, Wong KT, Antonio GE, *et al.* Severe acute respiratory syndrome: correlation between clinical outcome and radiologic features. *Radiology* 2004; 233: 579–585.
75. Pitzer VE, Leung GM, Lipstich M. Estimating variability in the transmission of severe acute respiratory syndrome to household contacts in Hong Kong, China. *Am J Epidemiol* 2007; 166: 355–363.
76. Poon LL, Chan KH, Wong OK, *et al.* Early diagnosis of SARS coronavirus infection by real time RT-PCR. *J Clin Virol* 2003; 28: 233–238.
77. Grant PR, Garson JA, Teddar RS, *et al.* Detection of SARS coronavirus in plasma by real-time RT-PCR. *N Engl J Med* 2003; 349: 2468–2469.

78. Ng EK, Hui DS, Chan KC, *et al.* Quantitative analysis and prognostic implication of SARS coronavirus in the plasma and serum of patients with severe acute respiratory syndrome. *Clin Chem* 2003; 49: 1976–1980.
79. Ng EK, Ng PC, Hon KL, *et al.* Serial analysis of the plasma concentration of SARS coronavirus RNA in pediatric patients with severe acute respiratory syndrome. *Clin Chem* 2003; 49: 2085–2088.
80. Lee N, Chan PK, Ip M, *et al.* Anti-SARS-CoV IgG response in relation to disease severity of severe acute respiratory syndrome. *J Clin Virol* 2006; 35: 179–184.
81. Tang F, Quan Y, Xin ZT, *et al.* Lack of peripheral memory B cell responses in recovered patients with severe acute respiratory syndrome: a six-year follow-up study. *J Immunol* 2011; 186: 7264–7268.
82. Wong RS, Wu A, To KF, *et al.* Haematological manifestations in patients with severe acute respiratory syndrome: retrospective analysis. *Br Med J* 2003; 326: 1358–1362.
83. Wong WM, Ho JC, Hung IF, *et al.* Temporal patterns of hepatic dysfunction and disease severity in patients with SARS. *JAMA* 2003; 290: 2663–2665.
84. Antonio GE, Ooi CG, Wong KT, *et al.* Radiographic-clinical correlation in severe acute respiratory syndrome: study of 1373 patients in Hong Kong. *Radiology* 2005; 237: 1081–1090.
85. Wong KT, Antonio GE, Hui DS, *et al.* Thin section CT of severe acute respiratory syndrome: evaluation of 73 patients exposed to or with the disease. *Radiology* 2003; 228: 395–400.
86. Joynt GM, Antonio GE, Lam P, *et al.* Late-stage adult respiratory distress syndrome caused by severe acute respiratory syndrome: abnormal findings at thin-section CT. *Radiology* 2004; 230: 339–346.
87. Gomersall CD, Joynt GM, Lam P, *et al.* Short-term outcome of critically ill patients with severe acute respiratory syndrome. *Intensive Care Med* 2004; 30: 381–387.
88. Shek CC, Ng PC, Fung GP, *et al.* Infants born to mothers with severe acute respiratory syndrome. *Pediatrics* 2003; 112: e254–e256.
89. Sung JJ, Wu A, Joynt GM, *et al.* Severe acute respiratory syndrome: report of treatment and outcome after a major outbreak. *Thorax* 2004; 59: 414–420.
90. Cinatl J, Morgenstern B, Bauer G, *et al.* Glycyrrhizin, an active component of liquorice roots, and replication of SARS-associated coronavirus. *Lancet* 2003; 361: 2045–2046.
91. Chu CM, Cheng VC, Hung IF, *et al.* Role of lopinavir/ritonavir in the treatment of SARS: initial virological and clinical findings. *Thorax* 2004; 59: 252–256.
92. Stroher U, DiCaro A, Li Y, *et al.* Severe acute respiratory syndrome-related coronavirus is inhibited by interferon-a. *J Infect Dis* 2004; 189: 1164–1167.
93. Tan EL, Ooi EE, Lin CY, *et al.* Inhibition of SARS coronavirus infection *in vitro* with clinically approved antiviral drugs. *Emerg Infect Dis* 2004; 10: 581–586.
94. Cinatl J, Morgenstern B, Bauer G, *et al.* Treatment of SARS with human interferons. *Lancet* 2003; 362: 293–294.
95. Sui J, Li W, Murakami A, *et al.* Potent neutralization of severe acute respiratory syndrome (SARS) coronavirus by a human mAb to S1 protein that blocks receptor association. *Proc Natl Acad Sci* 2004; 101: 2536–2541.
96. Chan KS, Lai ST, Chu CM, *et al.* Treatment of severe acute respiratory syndrome with lopinavir/ritonavir: a multicenter retrospective matched cohort study. *Hong Kong Med J* 2003; 9: 399–406.
97. Hurst M, Faulds D. Lopinavir. *Drugs* 2000; 60: 1371–1381.
98. Loutfy MR, Blatt LM, Siminovitch KA, *et al.* Interferon alfacon-1 plus corticosteroids in severe acute respiratory syndrome. A preliminary study. *JAMA* 2003; 290: 3222–3228.
99. Ho JC, Ooi GC, Mok TY, *et al.* High dose pulse *versus* non-pulse corticosteroid regimens in severe acute respiratory syndrome. *Am J Respir Crit Care Med* 2003; 168: 1449–1456.
100. So LK, Lau AC, Yam LY, *et al.* Development of a standard treatment protocol for severe acute respiratory syndrome. *Lancet* 2003; 361: 1615–1617.
101. Fisman DN. Hemophagocytic syndrome and infection. *Emerg Infect Dis* 2000; 6: 601–608.
102. Lai KN, Leung JC, Metz CN, *et al.* Role for macrophage migration inhibitory factor in acute respiratory distress syndrome. *J Pathol* 2003; 199: 496–508.
103. Tsang OT, Chau TN, Choi KW, *et al.* Coronavirus-positive nasopharyngeal aspirate as predictor for severe acute respiratory syndrome mortality. *Emerg Infect Dis* 2003; 9: 1381–1387.
104. Wang H, Ding Y, Li X, *et al.* Fatal aspergillosis in a patient with SARS who was treated with corticosteroids. *N Engl J Med* 2003; 349: 507–508.
105. Griffith JF, Antonio GE, Kumta SM, *et al.* Osteonecrosis of hip and knee in patients with severe acute respiratory syndrome treated with steroids. *Radiology* 2005; 235: 168–175.
106. Lee N, Allen Chan KC, Hui DS, *et al.* Effects of early corticosteroid treatment on plasma SARS-associated Coronavirus RNA concentrations in adult patients. *J Clin Virol* 2004; 31: 304–309.
107. Stockman LJ, Bellamy R, Garner P. SARS: systematic review of treatment effects. *PLoS Med* 2006; 3: e343.
108. Hui DS, Lee N, Chan PK. Adjunctive therapies and immunomodulatory agents in the management of severe influenza. *Antiviral Res* 2013; 98: 410–416.
109. Hui DS, Lee N. Adjunctive therapies and immunomodulating agents for severe influenza. *Influenza Other Respir Viruses* 2013; 7: Suppl. 3, 52–59.

110. Cheng Y, Wong R, Soo YO, *et al.* Use of convalescent plasma therapy in SARS patients in Hong Kong. *Eur J Clin Microbiol Infect Dis* 2005; 24: 44–46.
111. Soo Y, Cheng Y, Wong R, *et al.* Retrospective comparison of convalescent plasma with continuing high-dose methylprednisolone treatment in SARS patients. *Clin Microbiol Infect* 2004; 10: 676–678.
112. Mair-Jenkins J, Saavedra-Campos M, Baillie JK, *et al.* The effectiveness of convalescent plasma and hyperimmune immunoglobulin for the treatment of severe acute respiratory infections of viral etiology: a systematic review and exploratory meta-analysis. *J Infect Dis* 2015; 211: 80–90.
113. Li J, Ulitzky L, Silberstein E, *et al.* Immunogenicity and protection efficacy of monomeric and trimeric recombinant SARS coronavirus spike protein subunit vaccine candidates. *Viral Immunol* 2013; 26: 126–132.
114. ter Meulen J, van den Brink EN, Poon LL, *et al.* Human monoclonal antibody combination against SARS coronavirus: synergy and coverage of escape mutants. *PLoS Med* 2006; 3: e237.
115. Chan MH, Wong VW, Wong CK, *et al.* Serum LD1 isoenzyme and blood lymphocyte subsets as prognostic indicators for severe acute respiratory syndrome. *J Intern Med* 2004; 255: 512–518.
116. Gao W, Tamin A, Soloff A, *et al.* Effects of a SARS-associated coronavirus vaccine in monkeys. *Lancet* 2003; 362: 1895–1896.
117. Zhao P, Ke JS, Qin ZL, *et al.* DNA vaccine of SARS-CoV S gene induces antibody response in mice. *Acta Biochim et Biophysica Sinica* 2004; 36: 37–41.
118. Yang ZY, Kong WP, Huang Y, *et al.* A DNA vaccine induces SARS coronavirus neutralization and protective immunity in mice. *Nature* 2004; 428: 561–564.
119. Ho TY, Wu SL, Cheng SE, *et al.* Antigenicity and receptor-binding ability of recombinant SARS coronavirus spike protein. *Biochem Biophys Res Commun* 2004; 313: 938–947.
120. Choy WY, Lin SG, Chan PK, *et al.* Synthetic peptide studies on the severe acute respiratory syndrome (SARS) coronavirus spike glycoprotein: perspective for SARS vaccine development. *Clin Chem* 2004; 50: 1036–1042.
121. Zhong N. Management and prevention of SARS in China. *Philos Trans R Soc Lond B Biol Sci* 2004; 359: 1115–1116.
122. Ho PL, Tang XP, Seto WH. SARS: hospital infection control and admission strategies. *Respirol* 2003; 8: S41–S45.
123. Gopalakrishna G, Choo P, Leo YS, *et al.* SARS transmission and hospital containment. *Emerg Infect Dis* 2004; 10: 395–400.
124. CDC. SARS supplement I: infection control in healthcare, home and community settings. www.cdc.gov/sars/guidance/i-infection/downloads/i-infection-full.pdf Date last accessed: January 10, 2016. Date last updated: January 8, 2004.
125. Seto WH, Tsang D, Yung RW, *et al.* Effectiveness of precautions against droplets and contact in prevention of nosocomial transmission of severe acute respiratory syndrome (SARS). *Lancet* 2003; 361: 1519–1520.
126. Lau JT, Fung KS, Wong TW, *et al.* SARS transmission among hospital workers in Hong Kong. *Emerg Infect Dis* 2004; 10: 280–286.
127. Yu IT, Xie ZH, Tsoi KK, *et al.* Why did outbreaks of severe acute respiratory syndrome occur in some hospital wards but not in others? *Clin Infect Dis* 2007; 44: 1017–1025.
128. Tran K, Cimon K, Severn M, *et al.* Aerosol generating procedures and risk of transmission of acute respiratory infections to healthcare workers: a systematic review. *PLoS One* 2012; 7: e35797.
129. WHO. Severe acute respiratory syndrome (SARS) in Singapore – update 2. www.who.int/csr/don/2003_09_24/en/. Date last accessed: January 10, 2016. Date last updated: September 24, 2003.
130. WHO. Severe acute respiratory syndrome (SARS) in Taiwan, China. www.who.int/csr/don/2003_12_17/en/. Date last accessed: January 10, 2016. Date last updated: December 17, 2003.
131. Menachery VD, Yount BL Jr, Debbink K, *et al.* A SARS-like cluster of circulating bat coronaviruses shows potential for human emergence. *Nat Med* 2015; 21: 1508–1513.

Disclosures: None declared.

Chapter 2

Middle East respiratory syndrome coronavirus

Hasan M. Al-Dorzi[1], Maria D. Van Kerkhove[2], J.S. Malik Peiris[3] and Yaseen M. Arabi[1]

Since June 2012, MERS-CoV has been reported in more than 1600 individuals, some of whom have developed severe acute respiratory illness and multiorgan dysfunction. Most reported cases in Saudi Arabia have occurred as community-acquired sporadic infections and from human-to-human transmission in healthcare facilities. Cases in countries outside the Arabian Peninsula have been linked to travel to the Arabian Peninsula. Transmission from dromedary camels has been identified in several primary infections with MERS-CoV, with some of these leading to clusters of human-to-human transmissions, especially within healthcare facilities. The case-fatality rate in reported cases approaches 35%, but this does not take into account milder cases or asymptomatic infections that remain unrecognised. Strict adherence to infection prevention and control practices in healthcare is pivotal in preventing transmission in healthcare settings. At present, there is no specific therapy of proven effectiveness against MERS-CoV, and treatment is largely supportive. Further epidemiological studies and trials on potential therapies are needed for a better understanding and management of this disease.

MERS-CoV is a recently recognised virus that can lead to severe acute respiratory illness with multiorgan dysfunction. It is a CoV related to SARS-CoV. Although the spread of SARS was contained within a year, cases of MERS-CoV continue to occur, making it an ongoing public health threat in the Middle East and globally. This chapter summarises the current knowledge regarding the epidemiology, virology, pathogenesis, clinical manifestations, diagnosis and management of MERS-CoV infections.

Virology

MERS-CoV belongs to the genus *Coronavirus* within the family *Coronaviridae*, comprising enveloped, single-stranded RNA viruses [1], which can infect animals and humans, leading to illnesses ranging from the common cold to severe respiratory illnesses [1]. SARS-CoV, a beta-CoV of the B lineage that uses angiotensin-converting enzyme 2 as its cellular receptor [2, 3], caused a global outbreak in 2002–2003, leading to 8096 confirmed cases and 774 deaths in 29 countries or areas [4]. MERS-CoV is also a beta-CoV but of the C lineage.

[1]Intensive Care Dept, King Saud bin Abdulaziz University for Health Sciences and King Abdullah International Medical Research Center, King Abdulaziz Medical City, Riyadh, Saudi Arabia. [2]Center for Global Health, Institut Pasteur, Paris, France. [3]School of Public Health, Li Ka Shing Faculty of Medicine, Hong Kong SAR, China.

Correspondence: Yaseen M. Arabi, Intensive Care Dept, King Saud bin Abdulaziz University for Health Sciences, King Abdulaziz Medical City, P.O. Box 22490, Riyadh 11426, Saudi Arabia. E-mail: arabi@ngha.med.sa

 Print ISBN: 978-1-84984-069-9. Online ISBN: 978-1-84984-070-5. Print ISSN: 2312-508X. Online ISSN: 2312-5098.

Epidemiology

The epidemiology of MERS-CoV is characterised by occasional zoonotic transmission events, sometimes followed by outbreaks within healthcare settings. MERS-CoV was first isolated from a fatal case of severe pneumonia in Jeddah, Saudi Arabia, in June 2012 [5]. Subsequently, it was linked to a nosocomial cluster of respiratory illnesses in Jordan that occurred in March 2012 [6]. As of 23 January 2016, the World Health Organization (WHO) has reported 1626 laboratory-confirmed cases and 586 (36.0%) related deaths [7]. These cases have been reported from 26 countries, but initial zoonotic transmission from dromedary camels to humans has so far been reported only within the Arabian Peninsula. The majority (~75%) of cases have been reported from Saudi Arabia [7], where numerous clusters have occurred in healthcare settings across the country, including in Al Ahsa (April–May 2013) [8], Jeddah (April–May 2014) [9] and Riyadh (August–September 2015) [7, 10]. Hospital-acquired MERS cases represent 45% of all MERS cases, with 12% occurring in healthcare workers [11]. Patients with MERS acquired in the Middle East have sometimes travelled to and been diagnosed in Europe, North America, Africa and Asia, sometimes giving rise to secondary transmission within these countries [12, 13]. In May 2015, an outbreak in the Republic of Korea was the result of the delayed diagnosis of an infected patient who had returned after travelling to multiple Arabian Gulf countries [14]. Human-to-human and healthcare-associated transmission subsequently led to 186 MERS cases and 38 deaths [14]. The last reported new case in the Republic of Korea was on 4 July 2015 [15]. Analysis of disease clusters has suggested secondary and tertiary transmission, with some clusters attributed to superspreading events in some hospitals [16]. SARS-CoV has also led to several hospital outbreaks [17–20], but, in contrast to MERS, human-to-human transmission in SARS was more sustained, with an R_0 value (expected number of secondary infectious cases generated by an average infectious case in an entirely susceptible population) of 2.2–3.7 [21, 22].

In Saudi Arabia, it is recommended that severe pneumonia cases are investigated for MERS-CoV. In the 2013 Hajj pilgrimage season, none of 38 pilgrims with severe community-acquired pneumonia tested positive for MERS-CoV [23]. Among 5235 adult pilgrims from 22 countries screened using nasopharyngeal samples, none had MERS-CoV [24]. Several studies were performed on returning travellers from Saudi Arabia to different countries and did not document MERS-CoV infection; for example, during 2013–2014, in California, USA, 54 returning travellers from Saudi Arabia were investigated for MERS-CoV and none was positive [25], while in Austria, none of seven pilgrims returning from the 2014 Hajj with acute respiratory illnesses tested positive for MERS-CoV [26].

The presence of MERS-CoV has been tested in several animal species, and so far has been detected only in dromedary camels [27]. MERS-CoVs detected in dromedaries have some genetic diversity, with clades A and B being reported from the Arabian Peninsula, while more diverse non-A/non-B lineages have been reported in Africa [28]. Recent viruses infecting humans in the Arabian Peninsula have been clade B viruses. In 2014, a recombinant lineage emerged and become dominant in the Arabian Peninsula, resulting in the human outbreaks in 2015. Dromedaries are therefore an important natural host for the maintenance and diversification of MERS-CoV and appear to be the major source of zoonotic human infection [29].

The natural reservoir of MERS-CoV is still unknown, but bats may be one possible reservoir for the virus. However, accumulating evidence shows that dromedary camels are mainly responsible for animal-to-human transmission. The virus has been isolated from dromedary camels in the Arabian Peninsula and across North, East, West and Central Africa, but is not found in dromedary camels in Kazakhstan or in Bactrian camels in Mongolia or other countries, such as Japan [28, 30, 31]. However, only a minority of reported MERS human cases have reported direct camel exposure [32]. Detailed geographic and environmental analysis of the distributions of MERS-CoV cases in the Middle East suggests that higher temperatures and higher precipitation are associated with camel-to-human transmission [32]. The high viral loads in the upper respiratory tract of infected dromedaries suggest that transmission to humans occurs through close camel contact [33].

In a cross-sectional serosurveillance study of 10 009 healthy individuals from Saudi Arabia, 0.15% had evidence of positive MERS-CoV serology, suggesting that the number of mild or asymptomatic infections far outnumbers those that are recognised [34]. Seropositivity was more common in men than in women, in central than in coastal provinces, and in shepherds and slaughterhouse workers than in others [34]. However, in a study of 350 banked serum samples, collected at the start of an outbreak in July 2012 from individuals with self-reported domestic animal exposure (n=300) and controls (n=50) in Jazan Region, Saudi Arabia, a MERS spike protein pseudoparticle assay for the presence of MERS-CoV neutralising antibodies found that none of the samples was positive [35].

The risk factors for primary infection of MERS-CoV were analysed in a case–control study comprising 30 primary MERS-CoV cases reported from March to November 2014 in Saudi Arabia, with two to four controls matched by age, sex and neighbourhood for each case patient [36]. Using multivariable analysis, the authors demonstrated that direct dromedary exposure in the 2 weeks before illness onset was highly associated with MERS-CoV illness (adjusted OR 7.45, 95% CI 1.57–35.28), along with having diabetes (adjusted OR 6.99, 95% CI 1.89–25.86) or heart disease (adjusted OR 6.87, 95% CI 1.81–25.99) and current tobacco smoking (adjusted OR 6.84, 95% CI 1.68–27.94) [36].

Human-to-human transmission of MERS-CoV among close household contacts and family members of infected patients is infrequent [37], and sustained community-based transmission has not been reported. Human-to-human transmission within healthcare facilities is a key characteristic of MERS-CoV, and has been described for hospitalised patients and healthcare workers acquiring the disease [38–40]. The risk for secondary transmission from patients to household contacts was estimated at ~4% [41]. Healthcare-associated transmission has been attributed to many factors, most importantly delayed recognition and isolation of suspect cases, movement of infected patients prior to diagnosis, overcrowding in emergency rooms, and breaches in infection prevention and control practices [7]. Sequencing of MERS-CoV from the Jeddah outbreak and in Riyadh in April–June 2014 found evidence of two separate monophyletic chains of virus transmission, suggesting that these large outbreaks were caused by two separate zoonotic transmission events, each leading to transmission across multiple healthcare facilities [42, 43].

A study evaluating the stability of MERS-CoV under different environmental conditions found that the virus was more stable under low temperature/low humidity than higher temperature/higher humidity conditions [44]. Viable MERS-CoV could be recovered after 48 h at 20°C and 40% relative humidity [44]. During MERS-CoV aerosolisation, no decrease in stability was observed at 20°C and 40% relative humidity [44]. This raised the question of whether MERS-CoV may be transmitted *via* contact or fomite transmission due to prolonged environmental presence, especially in air-conditioned environments such as is found in modern hospitals [44]. MERS-CoV RNA has been detected in swabs taken from bed sheets, bedrails, intravenous fluid hangers, radiography devices, anterooms and air-ventilating equipment for up to 5 days following the last positive real-time RT-PCR result from patients' respiratory specimens [45]. The investigators isolated viable MERS-CoV from respiratory specimens of three patients obtained 18, 22 and 25 days after symptom onset [45].

Case definitions

The WHO defines a suspected MERS case as 1) an acute respiratory illness with fever and clinical, radiological or histopathological evidence of pulmonary involvement, together with a direct epidemiological link to a confirmed MERS-CoV case, and where a MERS-CoV test is unavailable, or where it is negative for a single inadequate specimen or is inconclusive; 2) an acute respiratory illness with fever and clinical, radiological or histopathological evidence of pulmonary involvement, and where the patient lives in or has travelled to the Middle East or to countries where MERS-CoV is known to be circulating in dromedary camels or where human MERS-CoV infections have recently occurred, and where a MERS-CoV test is inconclusive; or 3) an acute febrile respiratory illness of any severity, together with a direct epidemiological link to a confirmed MERS-CoV case, and where a MERS-CoV test is inconclusive [7]. A confirmed case is defined as a patient with laboratory-confirmed MERS-CoV infection, regardless of clinical signs and symptoms [7].

Clinical manifestations

The disease spectrum ranges from asymptomatic to rapidly progressive severe respiratory failure with multiorgan dysfunction. The incubation period of MERS is 2–14 days (median 5 days) [8, 46]. Severe cases usually occur in adults with chronic comorbidities, including diabetes mellitus, chronic cardiac disease, chronic lung disease, end-stage kidney disease and immunosuppression [47–49]. However, younger patients, including healthcare workers, sometimes suffer from severe disease [38]. Compared with SARS-CoV, MERS-CoV is more likely to affect older patients, men rather than women and people with comorbid illnesses. Healthcare-associated MERS-CoV infections were found to occur within the first week of the index case illness, while nosocomial transmission of SARS occurred mainly in the second week, probably due to the different timings of viral load peak [50]. Children have rarely been diagnosed with MERS, although it is possible that such infections are mild and therefore underdiagnosed [51]. Table 1 compares the clinical features of MERS with those of SARS.

The majority of critically ill MERS patients have fever (>65%), cough (>65%), dyspnoea (>65%) and gastrointestinal symptoms (32%) [47, 52]. Common laboratory abnormalities include leukopenia, lymphocytopenia and thrombocytopenia, and elevated serum creatinine, lactate dehydrogenase and liver enzymes [47, 52]. Initial chest radiographs are abnormal in most symptomatic patients, and findings range from minimal abnormality to extensive bilateral infiltrates [47, 52]. Computed tomography findings have included bilateral airspace opacities, predominantly in the subpleural and basilar lung regions, with more extensive ground-glass opacities than consolidation [53].

Rapid progression to hypoxaemic respiratory failure requiring intubation usually occurs within the first week after symptom onset [52]. The requirement for care in the ICU for hospitalised patients is frequent (45–70%) [39, 48], and is more common than in SARS (table 1) [54]. In one study at a single centre in Saudi Arabia (1 October 2012–31 May 2014), most MERS patients (65.7%) required intubation and mechanical ventilation [39]. In the univariate

Table 1. Comparison of the clinical features of MERS and SARS

Feature	MERS	SARS
Virus	Beta-CoV (lineage C) [1]	Beta-CoV (lineage B) [1]
Receptor	Dipeptidyl peptidase-4 [110]	Angiotensin-converting enzyme 2 [3]
Reservoir and intermediate hosts	Dromedary camels are a natural host [29]; the reservoir host remains undefined [111]	Probably bats and small mammals, such as civets [112]
Onset and duration	2012 and ongoing [7]	2002–2003 [4]
Cases n	1626# [7]	8096 [4]
Mode of transmission	Mostly droplets, fomites and aerosol; airborne cannot be excluded [44]	Mostly droplets, fomites and sometimes aerosol [81]
Human-to-human transmission	Yes (not sustained) [37]	Yes (sustained human-to-human transmission during the outbreak) [21, 113]
Mild or asymptomatic infections	Common [27]	Asymptomatic infection uncommon [114]; however, children and young adults had mild disease
Nosocomial transmission	45% of reported cases [11]	19–57% of reported cases [115]
Age of affected patients years	Median 62 [39], mean 56 [49]	Median 35–49¶ [4]
Male affected patients	65% [48]	47% [4]
Healthcare workers affected	12% [11]	19% [4]
Development of critical illness	45–89% [39, 49, 116]	20–32% [54]
Fatality rate	36.0% [7]	9.6% [4]
Critically ill	58–84% [39, 48, 52]	34–37%+ [57, 113]
Specific treatment	None proven to be effective	None proven to be effective

#: up to 23 January 2016; ¶: in series with >100 SARS cases; +: 28-day mortality.

analysis, factors associated with the requirement for ICU care were age ⩾65 years (OR 9.47, 95% CI 2.45–36.56), male sex (OR 3.05, 95% CI 1.05–8.84), higher age-adjusted Charlson comorbidity index (OR 1.35, 95% CI 1.11–1.65), bilateral pulmonary infiltrates on chest radiographs (OR 4.89, 95% CI 1.16–20.47), concomitant infections (OR 12.66, 95% CI 2.65–60.46) and serum albumin levels <35 $g \cdot L^{-1}$ at MERS diagnosis (OR 8.0, 95% CI 1.97–32.46) [39]. Severe neurological syndrome consisting of an altered level of consciousness, ataxia and focal motor deficits was reported in three critically ill MERS-CoV patients [55]. Brain magnetic resonance imaging showed widespread, bilateral hyperintense lesions on T2-weighted images in the white matter and subcortical areas of different brain regions [55].

The case-fatality rate of MERS-CoV infection is between 20% and 36% [7]. It should be noted, however, that mild and asymptomatic infections do occur and remain unreported, and thus the true case-fatality rate of MERS-CoV infection is likely to be much lower than this. However, the mortality rate of critically ill patients is higher (58–84%) [39, 48, 52]. In an observational study, 41 out of 49 (84%) MERS patients who required ICU care died [39]. Most (78.6%) had a progressive disease course until death [39]. On multivariate regression analysis, the presence of a concomitant infection (OR 14.13, 95% CI 1.58–126.09) and a low serum albumin level (OR 6.31, 95% CI 1.24–31.90) were associated with the need for ICU care [39]. Multivariate analysis found age ⩾65 years to be the only independent risk factor associated with increased mortality (OR 4.39, 95% CI 2.13–9.05) [39]. Viral load has been associated with mortality [56]. Critically ill SARS patients were shown to have high mortality, but the mortality was lower than that of MERS patients (table 1) [57]. Acute kidney injury (40.9%), hepatic dysfunction (31.4%) and cardiac arrhythmias (15.7%) are common complications of MERS [39]. An observational study of 12 critically ill cases found that vasopressors were used in 92% of patients, renal replacement therapy was performed in 58% and barotrauma occurred in 17% [52]. The median time from onset of symptoms to intubation was 4.5 days (range 0–33 days) [52]. The median ICU and hospital length of stay were 30 days (range 7–104 days) and 41 days (range 8–96 days), respectively, and 25% of patients had a tracheostomy [52]. The 28-day and 90-day mortality rates were 42% and 58%, respectively [52].

Pathogenesis

MERS-CoV uses the dipeptidyl peptidase-4 (DPP4) receptor, also known as CD26, to enter cells. The virus replicates in bronchial, bronchiolar, and type I and II alveolar epithelial cells, as well as in lung endothelial cells [58, 59]. MERS-CoV has been shown to infect human macrophages, dendritic cells and T-cells [60, 61]. It can induce cytokine dysregulation and T-cell apoptosis [60–62].

The highest viral loads have been detected in secretions from the lower respiratory tract, making these the specimens of choice for patients with MERS-CoV pneumonia [63, 64]. MERS-CoV patients may develop acute renal injury. As human kidneys heavily express the DPP4 receptor, direct viral infection is a potential mechanism, although this has not been confirmed directly [65]. Viral shedding has been documented in the urine and stool of infected patients [66].

The first autopsy of a MERS patient showed that MERS-CoV antigen was detected in pneumocytes and epithelial syncytial cells but not in extrapulmonary tissues [67]. The predominant finding in the lungs was diffuse alveolar damage [67]. In transgenic mice expressing human DPP4, MERS-CoV-infected lungs revealed mononuclear cell infiltration, alveolar oedema and microvascular thrombosis. The airways were generally unaffected [68]. Experimental infection of rhesus macaques with MERS-CoV led to multifocal mild-to-moderate interstitial pneumonia with exudative pathological changes [69]. Immunohistochemistry showed that type I and II pneumocytes and alveolar macrophages contained the viral antigen [69]. Other organs were not infected [69]. Marmosets infected with a high dose of MERS-CoV developed a more severe disease than rhesus macaques [70]. Histopathology demonstrated multifocal to coalescing, moderate to marked bronchointerstitial pneumonia around the terminal bronchioles and adjacent alveoli [70].

Laboratory diagnosis

The diagnosis of MERS-CoV is based on clinical criteria, exposure history and diagnostic findings [7]. Nevertheless, the clinical and radiological manifestations do not differentiate MERS-CoV infection from other causes of severe respiratory infections. Rapid and reliable laboratory diagnosis of suspected MERS cases is important for timely implementation of infection control practices and disease management. Currently, the diagnosis of MERS is confirmed by molecular testing. Real-time RT-PCR is used to target two regions of the viral genome: the upstream E protein, being more sensitive, is used for screening, while the open reading frame 1a (ORF1a) or ORF1b gene is used for confirmation [71]. Lower respiratory tract specimens have a higher viral load and thus provide better sensitivity than upper respiratory tract specimens [72]. The experience and expertise of laboratory personnel is important in collecting high-quality specimens for diagnosis. Avoidance of contamination and the specimen type and condition may affect the test result.

Reverse transcriptase loop-mediated isothermal amplification has been shown to exhibit a sensitivity similar to that of real-time RT-PCR for [73, 74]. It requires only a single temperature for amplification and can be completed in less than 1 h [73, 74]. Gene sequencing targeting the RNA-dependent RNA polymerase (present in all CoVs) and N gene (specific to MERS-CoV) fragments can be used for confirmation [71]. MERS-CoV can also be diagnosed by detecting seroconversion in two samples taken 2 weeks apart. ELISA can be used for screening, followed by an indirect immunofluorescence assay and neutralisation for confirmation [71]. A number of MERS-CoV-specific serological assays have been developed [71] and are currently being validated [75]. MERS-CoV can be cultured in Vero E6, Vero B4 and CaCo2 cells [71, 76]; however, performing viral culture requires specialised Biosafety Level 3 laboratories.

Susceptibility *in vitro* and *in vivo*

MERS-CoV has been found to be sensitive to IFN-α2b and ribavirin in Vero and LLC-MK2 cells *in vitro* [77]. However, the required concentrations of ribavirin were higher than can be achieved in humans. When combined, IFN-α2b and ribavirin at lower concentrations were effective in reducing MERS-CoV replication. In MERS-CoV-infected rhesus macaques, treatment with ribavirin and IFN-α2b led to reduced breathing abnormalities and a reduction in radiographic evidence of pneumonia compared with untreated animals [78]. There were also reduced levels of pro-inflammatory markers in the blood and lungs, a reduced viral load and less severe histopathological changes in the lungs [78].

Prevention of human-to-human transmission

Because of nosocomial transmission risk, strict implementation of infection prevention and control measures is important. Table 2 indicates suggested precautions to be taken during the care of MERS patients. For suspected cases, the WHO recommends droplet and contact precautions [79]. When performing an aerosol-generating procedure, such as aspiration or open suctioning of the respiratory tract, intubation, bronchoscopy and cardiopulmonary resuscitation, airborne precautions should be added [79]. The Centers for Disease Control and Prevention (CDC) recommends the application of droplet and standard precautions when caring for all patients with symptoms of ARI, and the isolation of a suspected or confirmed MERS-CoV case in an airborne infection isolation room [80]. If such a room is not available, the patient should be transferred as soon as possible to a facility where such a room is available [80]. Meanwhile, the patient should apply a facemask and be isolated in a room with its door closed [80]. Healthcare workers should adhere to standard contact and airborne precautions [80]. Hand hygiene should be performed appropriately, and personal protective equipment should be applied properly with respirators [80]. Eyes should be

Table 2. Suggested precautions during the care of patients with MERS-CoV infection

- Place the MERS patient in a negative-pressure room, or in an isolated single room if negative pressure is not available.
- Maintain a log of all persons entering the room.
- Restrict visitors as much as possible. Visitors should perform hand hygiene, apply contact and droplet precautions, and check on the patient from outside the room door. Visit duration should be limited to 10 min for each visitor. Those who have a febrile or respiratory illness should not be allowed into the unit.
- Limit the number of medical and nursing staff caring for the MERS patient.
- Use a combination of contact (hand hygiene, gowns, gloves) and airborne (fit-tested and fit-checked N-95 respirator) precautions and eye protection (goggles/face shield) when caring for the MERS patient.
- Clean room surfaces carefully and frequently with a hospital-grade disinfectant.
- Limit aerosol-generating procedures (*i.e.* administration of nebulised medications, suctioning, bronchoscopy).
- Avoid the use of noninvasive ventilation.
- Use closed-suctioning systems and high-efficiency particulate air filtration on the exhalation valve port in MERS patients receiving invasive mechanical ventilation.
- Instruct staff involved in the care of MERS patients not to report to work if symptoms develop and to visit employee health services for evaluation as soon as possible.

protected by goggles or a face shield. These precautions were shown in the SARS epidemic to prevent transmission of infection to healthcare workers [81].

Campaigns to educate the general public, and especially at-risk groups (*e.g.* men >60 years of age with underlying conditions), about good personal hygiene when in contact with dromedaries and the precautionary actions while eating camel meat or drinking its milk are important. Specific guidelines for the control and prevention of MERS-CoV transmission in healthcare settings to all staff in contact with patients, patient rooms or equipment should be in place. Additionally, hospitals should develop protocols to enhance surge capacity to be ready for a potential increase in the need to isolate patients with suspected or confirmed MERS-CoV infection.

Antiviral therapy and other potential treatments

To date, there is no effective specific treatment for MERS-CoV infection. Data on ribavirin, IFN and convalescent plasma in humans are limited [47]. A study in rhesus macaques found that a combination of IFN-α2b and ribavirin was associated with a reduction in MERS-CoV replication and an improved clinical outcome [78]. However, clinical studies on combined ribavirin and IFN have shown inconsistent results [82]. Convalescent sera from recovered patients might be a useful therapeutic intervention. A meta-analysis of 32 studies in patients infected with SARS-CoV or with severe influenza found that antibody treatment was associated with lower mortality compared with placebo or no treatment (pooled OR 0.25, 95% CI 0.14–0.45) [83]. However, the available studies were not randomised or adequately controlled [83]. Three studies from separate laboratories have reported the development of fully human neutralising monoclonal antibodies against MERS-CoV [84–86], but no clinical data are available so far [87]. Some camels in the Middle East have high titres of antibody to the virus. In mouse models, this antibody was found to be effective if delivered either prophylactically or therapeutically, but studies in humans are lacking [88]. Repurposed drugs with an *in vitro* anti-MERS-CoV effect, such as mycophenolic acid and anti-TNF agents, are not recommended outside clinical trials [89]. The feasibility, safety, and clinical and laboratory effects of convalescent plasma therapy remain under study [90].

Hence, at present, management of patients with MERS is primarily supportive. The WHO has issued guidance on MERS management, which focuses on appropriate infection control practices and organ support [79]. However, all these recommendations are based on evidence from general ICU studies, as specific data for MERS patients are lacking. Early invasive mechanical ventilation is indicated for significant respiratory distress or persistent hypoxaemia [79]. MERS patients with ARDS should be managed with a lung-protective ventilation strategy [91], targeting a tidal volume of 6 $mL \cdot kg^{-1}$ of predicted body weight, a plateau airway pressure of $\leqslant$30 cmH_2O, and arterial oxygen saturation of 88–95% or arterial oxygen tension (P_{aO_2}) of 55–80 mmHg. Moderate to severe ARDS cases (P_{aO_2}:F_{IO_2} (inspiratory oxygen fraction) <150 mmHg) are candidates for early prone positioning within 36 h of ARDS onset for at least 16 h per day [92] and early neuromuscular blockade using intravenous cisatracurium infusion for 48 h [93]. Extracorporeal membrane oxygenation may be an option for patients with refractory hypoxaemia [63, 94, 95]. The effect of corticosteroids on the outcome of MERS patients is unknown. However, their use has been associated with increased morbidity in SARS and severe influenza [96, 97]. Therefore, systematic corticosteroids are generally not advised, unless they are indicated for other reasons [79].

High-flow oxygen therapy, noninvasive ventilation and high-frequency oscillatory ventilation may be used with caution in MERS-CoV patients because of their ability to generate aerosols and the lack of effectiveness in ARDS, which frequently complicates MERS-CoV infection [98]. A systematic review of several observational studies found endotracheal intubation, noninvasive ventilation, tracheotomy and manual ventilation to be associated with an increased risk of ARI transmission to healthcare workers through aerosol generation [98]. Hence, strict infection prevention practices should be employed when they are performed.

Conservative fluid management is generally advocated in MERS patients with acute kidney injury and hypoxaemia in the absence of shock. Starting ultrafiltration at a lower level of fluid overload and early targeting of negative balance may be beneficial [99, 100]. Early trophic feeding for 7 days in ARDS patients [101] and permissive underfeeding for up to 14 days in mechanically ventilated patients [102] have been shown to have comparable outcomes to standard feeding. Underfeeding may be preferred during the prone position.

End-points for monitoring therapy

Respiratory shedding of MERS-CoV RNA may continue for >30 days in the majority of MERS-CoV-infected patients [103]. Discontinuation of isolation for confirmed MERS cases is suggested 7 days after complete resolution of MERS symptoms and after obtaining three consecutive negative lower respiratory tract samples that are >24 h apart [79].

Vaccines

Currently, there is no licensed MERS-CoV vaccine [104]. Developing effective vaccines against MERS-CoV has been the focus of many laboratories [104]. The S1 subunit of the virus, which contains the receptor-binding domain that mediates virus attachment to the DPP4 receptor, has been the focus of most immunisation strategies [105, 106]. An alternative vaccine regimen, tested in rhesus macaques and based on full-length spike glycoprotein DNA and a truncated S1 subunit glycoprotein, has been shown to elicit different neutralising antibodies with diverse mechanisms, showing promising protective results [107]. Vaccination of dromedary camels may help reduce zoonotic transmission, and a recent study has shown promising results [108]. However, the long-term effectiveness of such a vaccine strategy remains to be established.

Controversies, caveats or comments

While there is evidence for dromedary camels as a source of human infection, the mode of transmission remains unclear. It is not clear whether other animals can serve as the natural reservoir of MERS-CoV and as intermediate animal hosts for the virus. An animal model that accurately reflects the pathogenesis of the human disease is currently unavailable. Species such as Syrian hamsters, mice and ferrets, which are commonly used in animal studies, are not susceptible to MERS-CoV as they lack the DPP4 receptor [109]. Transgenic mice with human DPP4 and marmosets are animal models that have been used for testing of therapies and vaccines [70, 109].

Conclusion and future directions

MERS-CoV remains a significant threat to global public health. Infection with MERS-CoV is frequently severe and is associated with significant morbidity. The crude case-fatality rate of hospitalised cases is high (~35%), but this probably represents a skewed estimate because milder cases are not recognised. At present, the human disease is zoonotic in origin, sometimes followed by chains of transmission in humans, especially within healthcare settings. So far, such outbreaks have been contained by enhancing infection prevention and control measures. However, continued episodes of zoonotic transmission may provide the opportunity for the virus to acquire the capacity for sustained transmission in humans, as occurred with SARS in 2003. Our understanding of this virus continues to evolve, but large gaps exist in our knowledge of the modes of zoonotic transmission, clinical management and prevention. There is an urgent need for larger epidemiological and outcome studies and RCTs examining different therapeutic interventions.

References

1. Abdel-Moneim AS. Middle East respiratory syndrome coronavirus (MERS-CoV): evidence and speculations. *Arch Virol* 2014; 159: 1575–1584.
2. van Boheemen S, de Graaf M, Lauber C, *et al.* Genomic characterization of a newly discovered coronavirus associated with acute respiratory distress syndrome in humans. *MBio* 2012; 3: e00473-12.
3. Li W, Moore MJ, Vasilieva N, *et al.* Angiotensin-converting enzyme 2 is a functional receptor for the SARS coronavirus. *Nature* 2003; 426: 450–454.
4. World Health Organization. Summary of probable SARS cases with onset of illness from 1 November 2002 to 31 July 2003. www.who.int/csr/sars/country/table2004_04_21/en/ Date last accessed: January 23, 2016.
5. Zaki AM, van Boheemen S, Bestebroer TM, *et al.* Isolation of a novel coronavirus from a man with pneumonia in Saudi Arabia. *N Engl J Med* 2012; 367: 1814–1820.
6. Hijawi B, Abdallat M, Sayaydeh A, *et al.* Novel coronavirus infections in Jordan, April 2012: epidemiological findings from a retrospective investigation. *East Mediterr Health J* 2013; 19: Suppl. 1, S12–S18.
7. World Health Organization. Middle East respiratory syndrome coronavirus (MERS-CoV). www.who.int/emergencies/mers-cov/en/ Date last accessed: January 23, 2016.
8. Assiri A, McGeer A, Perl TM, *et al.* Hospital outbreak of Middle East respiratory syndrome coronavirus. *N Engl J Med* 2013; 369: 407–416.

9. Oboho IK, Tomczyk SM, Al-Asmari AM, *et al.* 2014 MERS-CoV outbreak in Jeddah – a link to health care facilities. *N Engl J Med* 2015; 372: 846–854.
10. Balkhy HH, Alenazi TH, Alshamrani MM, *et al.* Notes from the field: nosocomial outbreak of Middle East respiratory syndrome in a large tertiary care hospital – Riyadh, Saudi Arabia, 2015. *MMWR Morb Mortal Wkly Rep* 2016; 65: 163–164.
11. National Command and Control Center, Ministry of Health, Kingdom of Saudi Arabia. MERS-CoV Weekly Monitor. Vol 1, issue 1. October 27, 2015. www.moh.gov.sa/en/CCC/Pages/Weekly-Monitor.aspx Date last accessed: November 17, 2015.
12. Mailles A, Blanckaert K, Chaud P, *et al.* First cases of Middle East respiratory syndrome coronavirus (MERS-CoV) infections in France, investigations and implications for the prevention of human-to-human transmission, France, May 2013. *Euro Surveill* 2013; 18: 20502.
13. Bialek SR, Allen D, Alvarado-Ramy F, *et al.* First confirmed cases of Middle East respiratory syndrome coronavirus (MERS-CoV) infection in the United States, updated information on the epidemiology of MERS-CoV infection, and guidance for the public, clinicians, and public health authorities – May 2014. *MMWR Morb Mortal Wkly Rep* 2014; 63: 431–436.
14. Korea Centers for Disease Control and Prevention. Middle East respiratory syndrome coronavirus outbreak in the Republic of Korea, 2015. *Osong Public Health Res Perspect* 2015; 6: 269–278.
15. World Health Organization. Middle East respiratory syndrome coronavirus (MERS-CoV) – Republic of Korea. www.who.int/csr/don/25-october-2015-mers-korea/en/ Date last accessed: March 4, 2016.
16. Kucharski AJ, Althaus CL. The role of superspreading in Middle East respiratory syndrome coronavirus (MERS-CoV) transmission. *Euro Surveill* 2015; 20: 21167.
17. Goh KT, Cutter J, Heng BH, *et al.* Epidemiology and control of SARS in Singapore. *Ann Acad Med Singapore* 2006; 35: 301–316.
18. Varia M, Wilson S, Sarwal S, *et al.* Investigation of a nosocomial outbreak of severe acute respiratory syndrome (SARS) in Toronto, Canada. *CMAJ* 2003; 169: 285–292.
19. McDonald LC, Simor AE, Su IJ, *et al.* SARS in healthcare facilities, Toronto and Taiwan. *Emerg Infect Dis* 2004; 10: 777–781.
20. Leung GM, Hedley AJ, Ho LM, *et al.* The epidemiology of severe acute respiratory syndrome in the 2003 Hong Kong epidemic: an analysis of all 1755 patients. *Ann Intern Med* 2004; 141: 662–673.
21. Lee N, Hui D, Wu A, *et al.* A major outbreak of severe acute respiratory syndrome in Hong Kong. *N Engl J Med* 2003; 348: 1986–1994.
22. Lipsitch M, Cohen T, Cooper B, *et al.* Transmission dynamics and control of severe acute respiratory syndrome. *Science* 2003; 300: 1966–1970.
23. Memish ZA, Almasri M, Turkestani A, *et al.* Etiology of severe community-acquired pneumonia during the 2013 Hajj – part of the MERS-CoV surveillance program. *Int J Infect Dis* 2014; 25: 186–190.
24. Memish ZA, Assiri A, Almasri M, *et al.* Prevalence of MERS-CoV nasal carriage and compliance with the Saudi health recommendations among pilgrims attending the 2013 Hajj. *J Infect Dis* 2014; 210: 1067–1072.
25. Shahkarami M, Yen C, Glaser C, *et al.* Laboratory testing for Middle East respiratory syndrome coronavirus, California, USA, 2013–2014. *Emerg Infect Dis* 2015; 21: 1664–1666.
26. Aberle JH, Popow-Kraupp T, Kreidl P, *et al.* Influenza A and B viruses but not MERS-CoV in Hajj pilgrims, Austria, 2014. *Emerg Infect Dis* 2015; 21: 726–727.
27. Deem SL, Fevre EM, Kinnaird M, *et al.* Serological evidence of MERS-CoV antibodies in dromedary camels (*Camelus dromedaries*) in Laikipia County, Kenya. *PLoS One* 2015; 10: e0140125.
28. Chu DK, Oladipo JO, Perera RA, *et al.* Middle East respiratory syndrome coronavirus (MERS-CoV) in dromedary camels in Nigeria, 2015. *Euro Surveill* 2015; 20: 30086.
29. Sabir JS, Lam TT, Ahmed MM, *et al.* Co-circulation of three camel coronavirus species and recombination of MERS-CoVs in Saudi Arabia. *Science* 2016; 351: 81–84.
30. Shirato K, Azumano A, Nakao T, *et al.* Middle East respiratory syndrome coronavirus infection not found in camels in Japan. *Jpn J Infect Dis* 2015; 68: 256–258.
31. Chan SM, Damdinjav B, Perera RA, *et al.* Absence of MERS-coronavirus in Bactrian camels, Southern Mongolia, November 2014. *Emerg Infect Dis* 2015; 21: 1269–1271.
32. Reeves T, Samy AM, Peterson AT. MERS-CoV geography and ecology in the Middle East: analyses of reported camel exposures and a preliminary risk map. *BMC Res Notes* 2015; 8: 801.
33. Azhar EI, El-Kafrawy SA, Farraj SA, *et al.* Evidence for camel-to-human transmission of MERS coronavirus. *N Engl J Med* 2014; 370: 2499–2505.
34. Müller MA, Meyer B, Corman VM, *et al.* Presence of Middle East respiratory syndrome coronavirus antibodies in Saudi Arabia: a nationwide, cross-sectional, serological study. *Lancet Infect Dis* 2015; 15: 629.
35. Memish ZA, Alsahly A, Masri MA, *et al.* Sparse evidence of MERS-CoV infection among animal workers living in Southern Saudi Arabia during 2012. *Influenza Other Respir Viruses* 2015; 9: 64–67.

36. Alraddadi BM, Watson JT, Almarashi A, *et al.* Risk factors for primary Middle East respiratory syndrome coronavirus illness in humans, Saudi Arabia, 2014. *Emerg Infect Dis* 2016; 22: 49–55.
37. Memish ZA, Zumla AI, Al-Hakeem RF, *et al.* Family cluster of Middle East respiratory syndrome coronavirus infections. *N Engl J Med* 2013; 368: 2487–2494.
38. Memish ZA, Zumla AI, Assiri A. Middle East respiratory syndrome coronavirus infections in health care workers. *N Engl J Med* 2013; 369: 884–886.
39. Saad M, Omrani AS, Baig K, *et al.* Clinical aspects and outcomes of 70 patients with Middle East respiratory syndrome coronavirus infection: a single-center experience in Saudi Arabia. *Int J Infect Dis* 2014; 29: 301–306.
40. Ben Embarek PK, Van Kerkhove MD. Middle East respiratory syndrome coronavirus (MERS-CoV): current situation 3 years after the virus was first identified. *Wkly Epidemiol Rec* 2015; 90: 245–250.
41. Drosten C, Meyer B, Muller MA, *et al.* Transmission of MERS-coronavirus in household contacts. *N Engl J Med* 2014; 371: 828–835.
42. Drosten C, Muth D, Corman VM, *et al.* An observational, laboratory-based study of outbreaks of Middle East respiratory syndrome coronavirus in Jeddah and Riyadh, Kingdom of Saudi Arabia, 2014. *Clin Infect Dis* 2015; 60: 369–377.
43. Fagbo SF, Skakni L, Chu DK, *et al.* Molecular epidemiology of hospital outbreak of Middle East respiratory syndrome, Riyadh, Saudi Arabia, 2014. *Emerg Infect Dis* 2015; 21: 1981–1988.
44. van Doremalen N, Bushmaker T, Munster VJ. Stability of Middle East respiratory syndrome coronavirus (MERS-CoV) under different environmental conditions. *Euro Surveill* 2013; 18: 20590.
45. Bin SY, Heo JY, Song MS, *et al.* Environmental contamination and viral shedding in MERS patients during MERS-CoV outbreak in South Korea. *Clin Infect Dis* 2016; 62: 755–760.
46. Cauchemez S, Fraser C, Van Kerkhove MD, *et al.* Middle East respiratory syndrome coronavirus: quantification of the extent of the epidemic, surveillance biases, and transmissibility. *Lancet Infect Dis* 2014; 14: 50–56.
47. Alsolamy S. Middle East respiratory syndrome: knowledge to date. *Crit Care Med* 2015; 43: 1283–1290.
48. Al-Tawfiq JA, Hinedi K, Ghandour J, *et al.* Middle East respiratory syndrome coronavirus: a case–control study of hospitalized patients. *Clin Infect Dis* 2014; 59: 160–165.
49. Assiri A, Al-Tawfiq JA, Al-Rabeeah AA, *et al.* Epidemiological, demographic, and clinical characteristics of 47 cases of Middle East respiratory syndrome coronavirus disease from Saudi Arabia: a descriptive study. *Lancet Infect Dis* 2013; 13: 752–761.
50. Hui DS, Memish ZA, Zumla A. Severe acute respiratory syndrome vs. the Middle East respiratory syndrome. *Curr Opin Pulm Med* 2014; 20: 233–241.
51. Memish ZA, Al-Tawfiq JA, Assiri A, *et al.* Middle East respiratory syndrome coronavirus disease in children. *Pediatr Infect Dis J* 2014; 33: 904–906.
52. Arabi YM, Arifi AA, Balkhy HH, *et al.* Clinical course and outcomes of critically ill patients with Middle East respiratory syndrome coronavirus infection. *Ann Intern Med* 2014; 160: 389–397.
53. Ajlan AM, Ahyad RA, Jamjoom LG, *et al.* Middle East respiratory syndrome coronavirus (MERS-CoV) infection: chest CT findings. *AJR Am J Roentgenol* 2014; 203: 782–787.
54. Booth CM, Stewart TE. Severe acute respiratory syndrome and critical care medicine: the Toronto experience. *Crit Care Med* 2005; 33: Suppl., S53–S60.
55. Arabi YM, Harthi A, Hussein J, *et al.* Severe neurologic syndrome associated with Middle East respiratory syndrome corona virus (MERS-CoV). *Infection* 2015; 43: 495–501.
56. Feikin DR, Alraddadi B, Qutub M, *et al.* Association of higher MERS-CoV virus load with severe disease and death, Saudi Arabia, 2014. *Emerg Infect Dis* 2015; 21: 2029–2035.
57. Lew TW, Kwek TK, Tai D, *et al.* Acute respiratory distress syndrome in critically ill patients with severe acute respiratory syndrome. *JAMA* 2003; 290: 374–380.
58. Hocke AC, Becher A, Knepper J, *et al.* Emerging human Middle East respiratory syndrome coronavirus causes widespread infection and alveolar damage in human lungs. *Am J Respir Crit Care Med* 2013; 188: 882–886.
59. Chan RW, Chan MC, Agnihothram S, *et al.* Tropism of and innate immune responses to the novel human betacoronavirus lineage C virus in human ex vivo respiratory organ cultures. *J Virol* 2013; 87: 6604–6614.
60. Zhou J, Chu H, Li C, *et al.* Active replication of Middle East respiratory syndrome coronavirus and aberrant induction of inflammatory cytokines and chemokines in human macrophages: implications for pathogenesis. *J Infect Dis* 2014; 209: 1331–1342.
61. Chu H, Zhou J, Wong BH, *et al.* Productive replication of Middle East respiratory syndrome coronavirus in monocyte-derived dendritic cells modulates innate immune response. *Virology* 2014; 454–455: 197–205.
62. Chu H, Zhou J, Wong BH, *et al.* Middle East respiratory syndrome coronavirus efficiently infects human primary T lymphocytes and activates the extrinsic and intrinsic apoptosis pathways. *J Infect Dis* 2016; 213: 904–914.
63. Guery B, Poissy J, el Mansouf L, *et al.* Clinical features and viral diagnosis of two cases of infection with Middle East Respiratory Syndrome coronavirus: a report of nosocomial transmission. *Lancet* 2013; 381: 2265–2272.
64. World Health Organization. Laboratory testing for Middle East respiratory syndrome coronavirus: interim guidance. www.who.int/csr/disease/coronavirus_infections/mers-laboratory-testing/en/ Date last accessed: January 23, 2016.

65. Eckerle I, Muller MA, Kallies S, *et al.* In-vitro renal epithelial cell infection reveals a viral kidney tropism as a potential mechanism for acute renal failure during Middle East respiratory syndrome (MERS) coronavirus infection. *Virol J* 2013; 10: 359.
66. Drosten C, Seilmaier M, Corman VM, *et al.* Clinical features and virological analysis of a case of Middle East respiratory syndrome coronavirus infection. *Lancet Infect Dis* 2013; 13: 745–751.
67. Ng DL, Al Hosani F, Keating MK, *et al.* Clinicopathologic, immunohistochemical, and ultrastructural findings of a fatal case of Middle East respiratory syndrome coronavirus infection in the United Arab Emirates, April 2014. *Am J Pathol* 2016; 186: 652–658.
68. Li K, Wohlford-Lenane C, Perlman S, *et al.* Middle East respiratory syndrome coronavirus causes multiple organ damage and lethal disease in mice transgenic for human dipeptidyl peptidase 4. *J Infect Dis* 2016; 213: 712–722.
69. Yao Y, Bao L, Deng W, *et al.* An animal model of MERS produced by infection of rhesus macaques with MERS coronavirus. *J Infect Dis* 2014; 209: 236–242.
70. Falzarano D, de Wit E, Feldmann F, *et al.* Infection with MERS-CoV causes lethal pneumonia in the common marmoset. *PLoS Pathog* 2014; 10: e1004250.
71. Corman VM, Muller MA, Costabel U, *et al.* Assays for laboratory confirmation of novel human coronavirus (hCoV-EMC) infections. *Euro Surveill* 2012; 17: 20334.
72. Lee JH, Lee CS, Lee HB. An appropriate lower respiratory tract specimen is essential for diagnosis of Middle East respiratory syndrome (MERS). *J Korean Med Sci* 2015; 30: 1207–1208.
73. Shirato K, Yano T, Senba S, *et al.* Detection of Middle East respiratory syndrome coronavirus using reverse transcription loop-mediated isothermal amplification (RT-LAMP). *Virol J* 2014; 11: 139.
74. Bhadra S, Jiang YS, Kumar MR, *et al.* Real-time sequence-validated loop-mediated isothermal amplification assays for detection of Middle East respiratory syndrome coronavirus (MERS-CoV). *PLoS One* 2015; 10: e0123126.
75. Park SW, Perera RA, Choe PG, *et al.* Comparison of serological assays in human Middle East respiratory syndrome (MERS)-coronavirus infection. *Euro Surveill* 2015; 20: 30042.
76. Muth D, Corman VM, Meyer B, *et al.* Infectious Middle East respiratory syndrome coronavirus excretion and serotype variability based on live virus isolates from patients in Saudi Arabia. *J Clin Microbiol* 2015; 53: 2951–2955.
77. Falzarano D, de Wit E, Martellaro C, *et al.* Inhibition of novel β coronavirus replication by a combination of interferon-α2b and ribavirin. *Sci Rep* 2013; 3: 1686.
78. Falzarano D, de Wit E, Rasmussen AL, *et al.* Treatment with interferon-α2b and ribavirin improves outcome in MERS-CoV-infected rhesus macaques. *Nat Med* 2013; 19: 1313–1317.
79. World Health Organization. Clinical management of severe acute respiratory infection when Middle East respiratory syndrome coronavirus (MERS-CoV) infection is suspected: interim guidance. www.who.int/csr/disease/coronavirus_infections/case-management-ipc/en/ Date last accessed: January 23, 2016.
80. Centers for Disease Control and Prevention. Interim infection prevention and control recommendations for hospitalized patients with Middle East respiratory syndrome coronavirus (MERS-CoV). www.cdc.gov/coronavirus/mers/infection-prevention-control.html Date last accessed: January 23, 2016.
81. Seto WH, Tsang D, Yung RW, *et al.* Effectiveness of precautions against droplets and contact in prevention of nosocomial transmission of severe acute respiratory syndrome (SARS). *Lancet* 2003; 361: 1519–1520.
82. Al-Tawfiq JA, Momattin H, Dib J, *et al.* Ribavirin and interferon therapy in patients infected with the Middle East respiratory syndrome coronavirus: an observational study. *Int J Infect Dis* 2014; 20: 42–46.
83. Mair-Jenkins J, Saavedra-Campos M, Baillie JK, *et al.* The effectiveness of convalescent plasma and hyperimmune immunoglobulin for the treatment of severe acute respiratory infections of viral etiology: a systematic review and exploratory meta-analysis. *J Infect Dis* 2015; 211: 80–90.
84. Ying T, Du L, Ju TW, *et al.* Exceptionally potent neutralization of Middle East respiratory syndrome coronavirus by human monoclonal antibodies. *J Virol* 2014; 88: 7796–7805.
85. Jiang L, Wang N, Zuo T, *et al.* Potent neutralization of MERS-CoV by human neutralizing monoclonal antibodies to the viral spike glycoprotein. *Sci Transl Med* 2014; 6: 234ra59.
86. Tang XC, Agnihothram SS, Jiao Y, *et al.* Identification of human neutralizing antibodies against MERS-CoV and their role in virus adaptive evolution. *Proc Natl Acad Sci USA* 2014; 111: E2018–E2026.
87. Ying T, Li H, Lu L, *et al.* Development of human neutralizing monoclonal antibodies for prevention and therapy of MERS-CoV infections. *Microbes Infect* 2015; 17: 142–148.
88. Zhao J, Perera RA, Kayali G, *et al.* Passive immunotherapy with dromedary immune serum in an experimental animal model for Middle East respiratory syndrome coronavirus infection. *J Virol* 2015; 89: 6117–6120.
89. Zumla A, Azhar EI, Arabi Y, *et al.* Host-directed therapies for improving poor treatment outcomes associated with the Middle East respiratory syndrome coronavirus infections. *Int J Infect Dis* 2015; 40: 71–74.
90. Arabi Y, Balkhy H, Hajeer AH, *et al.* Feasibility, safety, clinical, and laboratory effects of convalescent plasma therapy for patients with Middle East respiratory syndrome coronavirus infection: a study protocol. *Springerplus* 2015; 4: 709.
91. Petrucci N, De Feo C. Lung protective ventilation strategy for the acute respiratory distress syndrome. *Cochrane Database Syst Rev* 2013; 2: CD003844.

92. Guerin C, Reignier J, Richard JC, *et al.* Prone positioning in severe acute respiratory distress syndrome. *N Engl J Med* 2013; 368: 2159–2168.
93. Papazian L, Forel JM, Gacouin A, *et al.* Neuromuscular blockers in early acute respiratory distress syndrome. *N Engl J Med* 2010; 363: 1107–1116.
94. Peek GJ, Mugford M, Tiruvoipati R, *et al.* Efficacy and economic assessment of conventional ventilatory support versus extracorporeal membrane oxygenation for severe adult respiratory failure (CESAR): a multicentre randomised controlled trial. *Lancet* 2009; 374: 1351–1363.
95. Davies A, Jones D, Bailey M, *et al.* Extracorporeal membrane oxygenation for 2009 influenza A(H1N1) acute respiratory distress syndrome. *JAMA* 2009; 302: 1888–1895.
96. Martin-Loeches I, Lisboa T, Rhodes A, *et al.* Use of early corticosteroid therapy on ICU admission in patients affected by severe pandemic (H1N1)v influenza A infection. *Intensive Care Med* 2011; 37: 272–283.
97. Stockman LJ, Bellamy R, Garner P. SARS: systematic review of treatment effects. *PLoS Med* 2006; 3: e343.
98. Tran K, Cimon K, Severn M, *et al.* Aerosol generating procedures and risk of transmission of acute respiratory infections to healthcare workers: a systematic review. *PLoS One* 2012; 7: e35797.
99. Ronco C, Ricci Z, De Backer D, *et al.* Renal replacement therapy in acute kidney injury: controversy and consensus. *Crit Care* 2015; 19: 146.
100. Han F, Sun R, Ni Y, *et al.* Early initiation of continuous renal replacement therapy improves clinical outcomes in patients with acute respiratory distress syndrome. *Am J Med Sci* 2015; 349: 199–205.
101. Rice TW, Wheeler AP, Thompson BT, *et al.* Initial trophic vs full enteral feeding in patients with acute lung injury: the EDEN randomized trial. *JAMA* 2012; 307: 795–803.
102. Arabi YM, Aldawood AS, Haddad SH, *et al.* Permissive underfeeding or standard enteral feeding in critically ill adults. *N Engl J Med* 2015; 372: 2398–2408.
103. Memish ZA, Assiri AM, Al-Tawfiq JA. Middle East respiratory syndrome coronavirus (MERS-CoV) viral shedding in the respiratory tract: an observational analysis with infection control implications. *Int J Infect Dis* 2014; 29: 307–308.
104. Zhang N, Jiang S, Du L. Current advancements and potential strategies in the development of MERS-CoV vaccines. *Expert Rev Vaccines* 2014; 13: 761–774.
105. Coleman CM, Liu YV, Mu H, *et al.* Purified coronavirus spike protein nanoparticles induce coronavirus neutralizing antibodies in mice. *Vaccine* 2014; 32: 3169–3174.
106. Du L, Kou Z, Ma C, *et al.* A truncated receptor-binding domain of MERS-CoV spike protein potently inhibits MERS-CoV infection and induces strong neutralizing antibody responses: implication for developing therapeutics and vaccines. *PLoS One* 2013; 8: e81587.
107. Wang L, Shi W, Joyce MG, *et al.* Evaluation of candidate vaccine approaches for MERS-CoV. *Nat Commun* 2015; 6: 7712.
108. Haagmans BL, van den Brand JM, Raj VS, *et al.* An orthopoxvirus-based vaccine reduces virus excretion after MERS-CoV infection in dromedary camels. *Science* 2016; 351: 77–81.
109. van Doremalen N, Munster VJ. Animal models of Middle East respiratory syndrome coronavirus infection. *Antiviral Res* 2015; 122: 28–38.
110. Raj VS, Mou H, Smits SL, *et al.* Dipeptidyl peptidase 4 is a functional receptor for the emerging human coronavirus-EMC. *Nature* 2013; 495: 251–254.
111. Corman VM, Ithete NL, Richards LR, *et al.* Rooting the phylogenetic tree of Middle East respiratory syndrome coronavirus by characterization of a conspecific virus from an African bat. *J Virol* 2014; 88: 11297–11303.
112. Li W, Shi Z, Yu M, *et al.* Bats are natural reservoirs of SARS-like coronaviruses. *Science* 2005; 310: 676–679.
113. Fowler RA, Lapinsky SE, Hallett D, *et al.* Critically ill patients with severe acute respiratory syndrome. *JAMA* 2003; 290: 367–373.
114. Leung GM, Lim WW, Ho LM, *et al.* Seroprevalence of IgG antibodies to SARS-coronavirus in asymptomatic or subclinical population groups. *Epidemiol Infect* 2006; 134: 211–221.
115. Lee N, Sung JJ. Nosocomial transmission of SARS. *Curr Infect Dis Rep* 2003; 5: 473–476.
116. Penttinen PM, Kaasik-Aaslav K, Friaux A, *et al.* Taking stock of the first 133 MERS coronavirus cases globally – is the epidemic changing? *Euro Surveill* 2013; 18: 20596.

Disclosures: H.M. Al-Dorzi reports receiving personal fees from Sanofi and grants from MSD, outside the submitted work.

Chapter 3

Interpandemic (seasonal) influenza

Sudhir Venkatesan[1], Rebecca J. Cox[2,3], Jonathan S. Nguyen-Van-Tam[1] and Puja R. Myles[1]

Influenza viruses belong to the family *Orthomyxoviridae* and are of four types: A, B, C and D. Types A and B cause measurable public health impact *via* regular epidemics in human populations. Influenza is seasonal in the temperate zones, but less so in the tropical and subtropical areas, where it can be found more or less all year round. A number of hypotheses have been proposed to explain the seasonality of influenza in temperate zones, but the exact causes remain unknown. Interpandemic influenza causes substantial morbidity and mortality globally, especially in the elderly ⩾65 years of age and in children <6 months of age. Influenza classically presents as an ARI with fever, and can potentially lead to a number of pulmonary and extrapulmonary complications. National and international guidelines for the control of interpandemic influenza include vaccination of population groups at risk of increased morbidity and mortality, and treatment with antiviral drugs in at-risk patients and in those who present or become severely unwell.

Although an influenza pandemic is recognised as a global public health emergency because of its potentially large impact in a relatively short period of time, the cumulative impact of recurrent interpandemic, or seasonal, influenza on morbidity and mortality is almost certainly greater [1, 2]. In addition the total burden of interpandemic influenza remains under-recognised, especially in children and in the developing world [3, 4]. Given that interpandemic influenza is clearly associated with excess mortality at the population level, it is of considerable public health importance; furthermore, the availability of moderately effective antiviral drugs and vaccines means that effective remedial action can be undertaken. In addition, interpandemic influenza serves as a blueprint for the future prevention and control of many other established and emerging respiratory viruses, where specific, targeted therapeutics are currently lacking.

Virology

Classification of influenza viruses

Influenza viruses are divided into four different types (A, B, C and D) by antigenic differences in their core proteins (matrix protein and nucleoprotein (NP)). Type A and B

[1]Division of Epidemiology and Public Health, Nottingham City Hospital, University of Nottingham, Nottingham, UK. [2]The Influenza Centre, Dept of Clinical Science, University of Bergen, Bergen, Norway. [3]Dept of Research and Development, Haukeland University Hospital, Bergen, Norway.

Correspondence: Jonathan S. Nguyen-Van-Tam, Room A28b, Clinical Sciences Building, University of Nottingham, City Hospital, Nottingham, NG5 1PB, UK. E-mail: jvt@nottingham.ac.uk

 Print ISBN: 978-1-84984-069-9. Online ISBN: 978-1-84984-070-5. Print ISSN: 2312-508X. Online ISSN: 2312-5098.

viruses cause significant illness in humans, resulting in regular outbreaks or epidemics, while influenza C virus causes a mild respiratory illness in humans, and influenza D has recently been identified in cattle [5]. Influenza A viruses can be further subdivided into subtypes based on the two major viral surface glycoproteins: haemagglutinin (HA) and neuraminidase (NA). So far, 18 variants of HA (H1–H18) and 11 variants of NA (N1–N11) have been identified in influenza A viruses, and most of the resulting subtypes (H/N combinations) are found in aquatic birds (H1–H16 and N1–N9). The influenza B viruses are divided into two lineages: B/Yamagata and B/Victoria [6]. Currently, the influenza A(H1N1) and A(H3N2) subtypes and both B lineages co-circulate continuously in humans.

In 1968, the influenza A(H3N2) subtype caused a pandemic, replacing the previously circulating A(H2N2) virus. A(H3N2) viruses have continued to circulate since this time, undergoing progressive and stepwise antigenic changes, with at least 14 antigenically distinct viruses found, which are often associated with higher mortality levels [7]. In 1977, the A(H1N1) subtype reappeared after a 20-year period without circulation, causing illness in children and young adults. This A(H1N1) subtype continued to co-circulate with the A (H3N2) subtype. In 2009, a novel triple reassortment influenza A(H1N1) virus derived from North American and Eurasian swine lineages caused the first pandemic of the 21st century [8]. This virus replaced the previously circulating seasonal A(H1N1) virus and has continued to circulate as a seasonal strain. Since the 1970s, two genetically distinct lineages of influenza B have circulated [9–11], and the recent introduction of quadrivalent influenza vaccines covers both lineages.

Nomenclature

In 1980, the World Health Organization (WHO) adopted revised guidelines for the nomenclature of influenza viruses [12]. Naming is undertaken according to: influenza type (A, B or C); host of origin (*e.g.* chicken, equine, swine), if non-human; geographical origin of the isolate; strain number; and year of isolation. For influenza A viruses, the subtype is added in parentheses, *e.g.* the human isolate of influenza A/Switzerland/9715293/2013 (H3N2).

Originally, influenza viruses were typed and subtyped using serological tests, but genetic characterisation of isolates now allows division of viruses into clades within a phylogenetic tree. For example, avian influenza A(H5N1) viruses are divided into clades and suborder clades according to their HA sequence [13].

Virus structure

The influenza viruses are members of the family *Orthomyxoviridae* and are negative-sense, single-stranded (ss) RNA viruses with a segmented genome. Influenza A and B viruses have eight gene segments and a similar virus structure, while type C virus has only seven RNA segments and a single glycoprotein called haemagglutinin esterase. The sizes of the genomic segments of influenza A virus vary from 890 to 2341 bp, encoding up to 17 proteins (table 1). The virus is pleomorphic, and the structure of the virion can be spherical or filamentous, with a diameter of 80–120 nm. The virus is enveloped, with a helical core ribonucleoprotein (RNP), consisting of ssRNA and the scaffolding protein, NP (figure 1) [19]. Three viral polymerase proteins (PB1, PB2 and PA) comprise the viral polymerase complex, and a single complex is bound to each RNP segment [17]. The matrix protein 1 (M1) surrounds the RNP, lining the inner surface of the viral envelope. The viral lipid bilayer or envelope is derived from the host cell plasma membrane upon budding of

Table 1. Influenza A genome segments

Virus segment	Nucleotides/ amino acids	Protein [ref.]	Protein copies per virion	Function
1	2341 nt/759 aa	PB2	30–60	Polymerase complex involved in virus replication
2	2341 nt/757 aa	PB1	30–60	Polymerase complex involved in virus replication
		PB1-F2		Induces apoptosis in infected cells
		N40 [14]		
3	2233 nt/716 aa	PA	30–60	Polymerase complex involved in virus replication
		PA-X		Endonucleolytic activity, modification of host immune response
		PA-N155 [15]		Probably role in virus life cycle
		PA-N182		Probably role in virus life cycle
4	1778 nt/566 aa	HA	500	Haemagglutinin, surface glycoprotein; binds cellular receptor; involved in release of viral ribonucleoprotein through fusion of the virus and endosome membrane
5	1565 nt/498 aa	NP	1000	Nucleoprotein, encapsulates RNA, type-conserved antigen used for typing A, B and C viruses
6	1413 nt/454 aa	NA	100	Neuraminidase, surface glycoprotein, sialidase enzyme; removes sialic acid from HA, aiding in cell entry and egress (prevents aggregation of virions)
7	1027 nt			
	M1 252 aa	M1	3000	Matrix protein
	M2 99 aa	M2	20–60	Ion channel integral membrane protein
		M42 [16]		Can replace M2
8	890 nt			
	NS1 230 aa	NS1		Host IFN antagonist
	NS2/NEP 121 aa	NS2	130–200	Nuclear export protein

nt: nucleotides; aa: amino acids; PA/PB1/PB2: polymerase proteins; HA: haemagglutinin; NP: nucleoprotein; NA: neuraminidase; M: matrix protein; NS: nonstructural protein. Reproduced and modified from [17] with permission.

the progeny virus and is composed of three integral membrane proteins: one transmembrane protein (the matrix protein 2 (M2)) and the two surface glycoproteins (HA and NA, in a ratio of approximately 5:1).

Virus life cycle

Figure 2 shows a simplified replication cycle of influenza A virus; the numbers in the text refer to the different phases in the life cycle. On the virus surface, the HA protein (figure 2: locus 1)

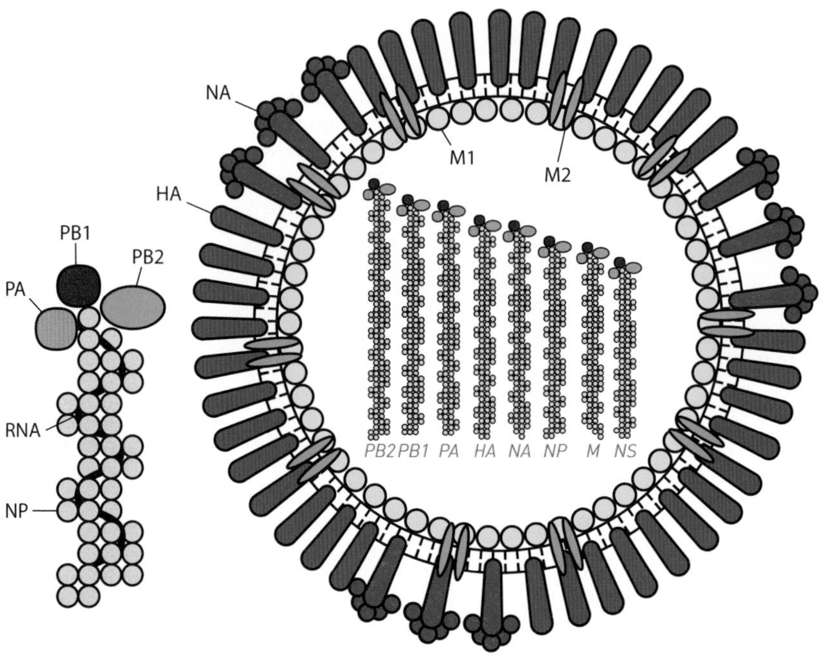

Figure 1. Structure of influenza A virus. NA: neuraminidase; HA: haemagglutinin; M: matrix protein; PA/PB1/PB2: polymerase proteins; NP: nucleoprotein; NS: nonstructural protein. Image provided by K.A. Brokstad (University of Bergen, Bergen, Norway). Reproduced and modified from [18] with permission.

contains the receptor-binding site, which binds to the virus receptor, *N*-acetyl neuraminic acid (sialic acid (SA)), on epithelial cells in the upper respiratory tract (locus 2). The virus enters the cell through receptor-mediated endocytosis (locus 3). In the low pH of the endosome, protons flow through the M2 ion channel, causing acidification of the interior of the virion, allowing the viral RNPs to dissociate from the M1 protein. The HA undergoes a conformational change, exposing a fusion peptide, and allowing fusion of the viral envelope with the endosomal membrane and subsequent release of the viral RNPs into the cytoplasm (locus 4). The RNPs are translocated to the nucleus, where they are transcribed into mRNA by the viral RNA polymerase complex (locus 5). The virus hijacks the cell, using the cell machinery to produce progeny virus. The viral RNA replicates using positive-sense complementary RNA to produce the viral RNA genome. The membrane proteins undergo post-translational modifications in the Golgi apparatus (locus 6). After cytoplasmic synthesis, the viral RNPs are assembled in the nucleus and thereafter transported to the cell surface (locus 7), where the virus assembles with the integral membrane proteins HA, NA and M2, and then buds off through the lipid membrane (locus 8). NA is important in the egress of the virus so that HA does not bind to receptors on the host cell. NA cleaves SA from complex carbohydrate chains and is the target for neuraminidase inhibitor (NI) drugs. Recent evidence has shown that influenza virus infectious cores (RNP and polymerase) can spread to neighbouring cells without extracellular budding [20].

The HA protein

HA is a homotrimeric integral membrane protein that radiates from the viral envelope. It is synthesised as a single polypeptide precursor (HA0), which is cleaved by host trypsin-like proteases into HA1 (the globular head) and HA2 (the stalk domain), which are linked

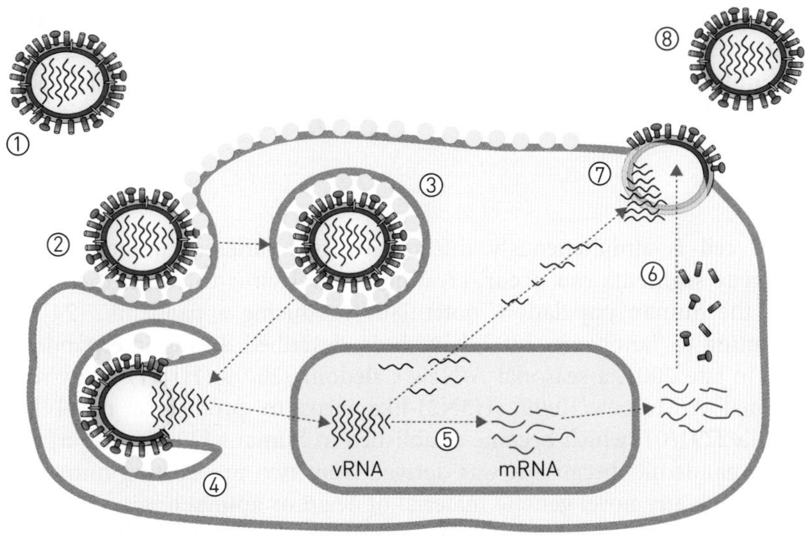

Figure 2. Replication cycle of influenza A virus. vRNA: viral RNA. Details about the locus numbers are provided in the Virus life cycle section of the main text. Image provided by K.A. Brokstad (University of Bergen, Bergen, Norway).

together by a disulfide bond [21]. Antibodies that bind to the globular head domain of HA neutralise the virus and inhibit virus entry into the host cell. The HA2 domain is highly conserved; it contains the conformation-dependent fusion peptide and forms the stalk domain, together with both the N and C termini of HA1. The highly conserved stalk can be used to divide influenza A viruses into two groups: group 1 (including H1, H2 and H5 viruses) and group 2 (including H3 and H7 viruses). Anti-stalk antibodies are broadly neutralising and can function in a number ways, including preventing infection by inhibiting cleavage of the HA0 precursor or inhibiting viral membrane fusion in the endosome, or by mediating antibody-dependent cellular cytotoxicity of the infected cell.

Influenza virus infection is mediated by the receptor-binding site on the HA protein binding to the SA receptor on a target cell. Human influenza viruses bind to SA linked by α-2,6 linkage; in humans, these receptors are found predominantly in the upper respiratory tract. Avian influenza viruses bind to SA with α-2,3 linkage, the receptors for which are expressed mainly in the alveoli of the lower respiratory tract in humans (reviewed in [22]). The human soft palate uniquely contains long-chain α-2,6-linked SA and has been shown to rapidly select transmissible α-2,6 SA-binding viruses from α-2,3-binding viruses [23]. Aquatic birds are the natural reservoir for influenza A viruses, and constitute a risk for the introduction of new influenza A subtypes into humans through zoonosis, as exemplified by the influenza A (H5N1) and A(H7N9) viruses.

Antigenic drift

In a process called antigenic drift, influenza viruses in humans continually undergo antigenic changes in their surface glycoproteins (HA and NA), resulting in escape of the host's acquired humoral immunity. Antigenic drift occurs because of the lack of accurate proofreading ability of the RNA-dependent RNA polymerase, resulting in point mutations in the viral genome and, in particular, mutations in the outer head of the HA protein, which give the novel virus a selective advantage. Once high levels of strain-specific antibodies are present in the population, the novel drifted virus exerts its selective advantage to become the predominant circulating strain. Antigenic drift is responsible for the annual interpandemic outbreaks of influenza; consequentially, the influenza strains in the seasonal vaccine require annual review, and frequently one or more of the components requires updating.

Antigenic shift

When a host cell is simultaneously infected by two different influenza A viruses, an exchange of gene segments can occur, creating a novel virus to which there is little or no immunity in the human population, potentially producing a pandemic [24]. Reassortant events, amounting to "antigenic shift", have been described during interpandemic periods. For example, in late 2001, a seasonal A/New Caledonia/20/99 (H1N1)-like virus reassorted with a seasonal A/Moscow/10/99 (H3N2)-like virus to produce a novel H1N2 virus, A/Saudi Arabia/2231/01, which became established in humans [25]. However, this virus did not produce a pandemic, because it was derived from two pre-existing human viruses and did not incorporate any novel genetic material of avian or animal origin.

Epidemiology

Timing and seasonality

Temperate regions

Influenza is distinctly seasonal in the temperate regions of the northern and southern hemispheres, with outbreaks typically occurring during winter [26, 27]. While one subtype of influenza A or B virus usually predominates in any given season, A(H1N1), A(H3N2) and two lineages of influenza B virus co-circulate to some extent, and mixed epidemics are periodically observed. In temperate zones of the northern hemisphere, influenza transmission generally occurs between November and early spring [28], and at much lower levels during the summer months [28]. The reciprocity of summer and winter seasons in the northern and southern hemispheres corresponds to an oscillation of influenza activity in the temperate regions across the equator [29].

The close correlation between winter and increased influenza transmission in temperate zones strongly suggests that seasonality may be related to environmental factors during winter, including lower temperatures and a decrease in solar radiation [27, 30]. It has also been argued that human behaviour and lifestyle changes during colder seasons, such as increased indoor crowding in small spaces with little ventilation, may be responsible for increased influenza activity during winter [29, 31, 32]. Another proposed mechanism for the seasonality of influenza relates to seasonal variations in virus survival. Low humidity is associated with longer virus survival in both aerosol form [33–35] and on steel surfaces [36], and decreased temperatures are known to cause an increase in the stability of influenza virus and improved survival through mechanisms linked to phospholipid ordering [37]. Studies performed in ferrets have demonstrated that influenza transmission occurred most efficiently at relative humidity (RH) levels between 20% and 35%. Transmission levels dropped at RH levels of 50%, but increased again at RH levels of 65%. No transmission was reported at RH levels of 80% [38–40].

Variations in host immunity may also play a role in the observed seasonality of influenza. In temperate regions, the low levels of solar radiation observed during winter could contribute to lower levels of vitamin D in the body [41, 42], resulting in reduced host immunity and increased susceptibility to influenza virus. The evidence from RCTs for the association between influenza and vitamin D is inconclusive, with one trial suggesting a protective effect of vitamin D supplements during winter on the incidence of influenza A in children [43] and another trial suggesting no association in adults [44]. Although it is possible that all of the above factors contribute to the seasonality of influenza, the precise reasons and mechanisms for this remain unclear [45, 46].

Tropical and equatorial regions

Compared with temperate regions, the epidemiology of influenza in tropical and equatorial regions has not been studied as extensively. However, the seasonality of influenza in tropical regions is not as marked [47], and there is generally background activity throughout the year [48]. In addition to year-round background activity, data from some tropical countries suggest two periods of increased influenza activity. A study from Hong Kong investigating reports of ILI from outpatient clinics between 1998 and 2006 reported two broad patterns of ILI: 5 years with semi-annual cycles with two peaks, one in winter and the other towards the end of spring; and 4 years with only one pronounced peak of influenza-like activity [49]. In a study in Thailand conducted between 1988 and 1995, influenza A and B viruses were isolated all year round, with 67% of cases occurring between June and October, coinciding with the rainy season, and a smaller peak in March [50]. Data from India showed influenza patterns similar to those observed in Thailand, with two peaks against year-round background influenza activity, with one of the peaks coinciding with the rainy season [51]. Like Thailand, Singapore has been observed to show two peaks of influenza activity, although the larger peak tends to occur during the warmer months between April and June, with a smaller peak in winter [52, 53]. Seasonal influenza patterns in Brazil occur in the form of a wave originating in the equatorial north of the country around March, which then sweeps southwards over approximately the next 3 months [54].

Diagnosis and surveillance of influenza

Influenza typically presents as an ARI. However, asymptomatic cases of influenza have been shown to account for at least one-half of all infections detected serologically [55–57]. Additionally, a number of other ARIs present with clinical features similar to influenza, making the use of laboratory techniques such as the PCR test or near-patient tests (NPTs) essential to establish an accurate diagnosis of influenza. Information on influenza virus activity during an epidemic, specifically the type and nature of virus in circulation, the impact of the influenza epidemic and detection of any unusual events, is crucial for healthcare workers and policy makers to inform antiviral treatment decisions, and for vaccine development and other epidemic mitigation measures [58].

In humans, surveillance of influenza broadly comprises two components: 1) clinical surveillance, necessary to track temporal and geographical patterns of illness and to identify any new clinical symptoms, and commonly maintained through electronic medical records from outpatient practices and hospitals linked to laboratory confirmation of influenza, as well as through internet surveys; and 2) virological surveillance, performed to determine the exact virus type and antigenic changes over time, assess vaccine effectiveness for circulating strains, identify antiviral resistance and potentially signal detection of a novel virus with pandemic potential.

Effective surveillance systems are central to epidemic and pandemic mitigation plans. The WHO has established a global network, called the Global Influenza Surveillance and

Response System (GISRS), comprising over 140 National Influenza Centres to test clinical specimens from around the world in order to monitor viral antigenicity, help identify strains and subsequently provide viral samples for vaccine development [59]. However, the principal goal of global influenza surveillance is to aid in advanced detection of the disease, so that the public health impact can be minimised [59]. The 2009 A(H1N1) pandemic exposed a number of gaps in worldwide influenza surveillance systems. Lack of data on severe disease in relation to past outbreaks in most countries, the absence of a global data-sharing mechanism and the lack of standardisation of data collection procedures were identified as the key shortcomings in existing surveillance systems [59]. Among the recommendations made by the WHO to address these shortcomings were: 1) adopting a global standard for minimal respiratory disease surveillance, and 2) integrating routine surveillance of SARIs into existing public health systems [59].

Burden of illness

Excess mortality

According to the WHO, 250 000–500 000 deaths and about 3–5 million cases of severe illness occur annually as a result of influenza [60]. While these estimates are based on an extrapolation of estimates from the USA, data from some tropical countries, such as Hong Kong, have reported mortality figures comparable to temperate countries [47]; however, in many developing countries, the burden of influenza is simply not known. Accurate ascertainment of the burden of illness due to influenza is difficult for a number of reasons. The clinical presentation of influenza is similar to other respiratory virus infections, and patients in hospitals with ARIs are not routinely tested for respiratory virus infection [61], making it difficult to fully attribute illnesses and deaths due to influenza. Additionally, influenza is known to cause secondary infections and to aggravate chronic conditions [62], making it even more challenging to assess the total burden of illness.

Conventionally, influenza-related mortality has been calculated by estimating the additional or excess mortality compared with the expected baseline mortality for winter. This concept of excess mortality was first described in 1847 [63] and was developed statistically by Serfling [64]. There have been numerous subsequent methodological enhancements [65–67], but the basic approach is still considered useful [68].

Attack rates

In order to correctly assess the impact of influenza on the community, it is important to consider longitudinal studies that, along with clinical surveillance, also record laboratory confirmation of influenza. Two cohort studies were performed in the USA: in Tecumseh, Michigan, between 1966 and 1971; and in Seattle, Washington, between 1965 and 1969, and between 1975 and 1979 [69, 70]. These studies investigated families with young children, using self-reported details combined with virus isolation and serological sampling [69, 70]. From 1966 to 1971 in Michigan, the annual population attack rate was 17% for type A influenza virus and 8% for type B influenza virus [70]. Over an overlapping period between 1965 and 1969 in Seattle, attack rates of 19% and 20% for influenza virus types A and B, respectively, were observed. The A(H1N1) influenza epidemic of 1978–1979 in Seattle showed an attack rate of 31%, but occurred almost entirely in children [69]. In 2014, Hayward *et al.* [57] published findings from the UK's first national-level influenza cohort study recruiting families from the community with RT-PCR testing, named the Flu Watch study. The Flu Watch study followed recruited families for 5 years between 2006 and 2011.

The dominant influenza virus strains observed were A(H3N2) in 2006–2007, seasonal A(H1N1) in 2007–2008, A(H3N2) in 2008–2009 and pandemic A(H1N1) in 2009–2011 [57]. The rate for PCR-confirmed influenza was 4% for each winter and 3% during the pre-pandemic phase, and increased to 5% during the pandemic. It was evident from the different sources of data that there was a noticeable variation in attack rates between seasons. However, attack rates in children were consistently highest in all three studies: 23% for children under 1 year of age in Michigan; 24% and 26% for types A and B, respectively, for pre-school children in Seattle; and similarly increased in the Flu Watch study [57, 69, 70]. These findings are in agreement with a number of other studies, suggesting that children play an important part in the rapid dissemination of influenza in the community [71, 72]. GLEZEN *et al.* [73] performed a prospective study in the Houston area in 1974–1976 and found that pre-school children were associated with an attack rate of 30%, but that the risk shifted to young adults as the epidemic progressed over time. Two distinct and divergent influenza B virus lineages (B/Yamagata and B/Victoria) have co-circulated since the mid-1970s [9–11]. Some clinico-epidemiological data have emerged recently, suggesting that B/Victoria infections predominate in young children, whereas B/Yamagata strains are more evenly age distributed [74, 75].

Risk groups

Increased susceptibility to influenza-related serious illness or death has been observed consistently in young children <6 months of age and the elderly ⩾65 years of age [76–80]. People with one or more of the following comorbidities are four to 10 times more likely to be admitted to hospital due to an influenza virus infection when compared with otherwise healthy people: asthma and any other chronic respiratory disease, immunosuppression, and renal, hepatic, cardiovascular, haematological, neurological or metabolic disease [81]. Adverse outcomes have also been reported in pregnant women infected with pandemic as well as with seasonal influenza virus. Pregnant women infected with influenza virus can experience decreased neonatal birthweight, prematurity, perinatal mortality and even death [82, 83]. A recent study, based on data from the USA, showed that morbid obesity (body mass index ⩾40 $kg \cdot m^{-2}$) was independently associated with an increase in the likelihood of hospitalisation by 4.7 times and an increase in the likelihood of death by 7.6 times, following 2009 A(H1N1) pandemic influenza virus infection [84].

Clinical manifestations

Influenza typically presents as an ARI with fever (>37.8°C), cough, sore throat and malaise [85], commonly defined as ILI. However, because the rate of asymptomatic influenza virus infection is so high and the spectrum of possible illness severity so broad, influenza virus cannot reliably be distinguished from other respiratory viruses based on clinical symptoms [86]. Nevertheless, during a known influenza epidemic (defined by high-quality surveillance data), the likelihood of ILI indicating influenza virus infection is quite high, with cough and fever having a positive predictive values of 79% for laboratory-confirmed influenza in some studies [87]. The clinical presentation of influenza virus-related illness in hospitalised patients tends to be more complicated. In hospitalised patients, the positive predictive value of ILI drops significantly to 23–50% [88]. Unexplained respiratory illness with other systemic complications in hospitalised patients therefore warrants an evaluation of possible exposure to influenza viruses, including evidence of local community transmission or recent travel to areas with active influenza outbreaks, coupled with laboratory investigations for a broad range of respiratory virus aetiologies.

Pulmonary complications

Of the many respiratory-tract-related complications associated with influenza A and B viruses, acute bronchitis is the most common complication in adults (seen in ~20% of patients) and otitis media with lower respiratory tract infection in children (seen in >25% of patients) [86]. Pneumonia is a significant complication of influenza, with influenza-related pneumonia accounting for ~18% of all community-acquired viral pneumonia identified in adults [89]. Although the available data are difficult to interpret, about one-quarter of all influenza virus infections seem to be complicated by secondary bacterial respiratory infection [90, 91], some of which presents as pneumonia. *Streptococcus pneumoniae* and *Staphylococcus aureus* are the most common causes of secondary bacterial pneumonia [92–94]. One study from Sweden estimated that invasive pneumococcal pneumonia increased by 12–20% after peaks in influenza activity [92]. For *S. aureus* coinfections, one retrospective study using US surveillance data reported that methicillin-resistant *S. aureus* (MRSA) accounted for >50% of *S. aureus* isolates [93]. *Haemophilus influenzae* and *Streptococcus pyogenes* are other pathogens less commonly associated with secondary bacterial pneumonia [94]. Secondary bacterial pneumonia accounts for nearly 25% of all influenza-related deaths [93, 95].

Systemic complications

Influenza has been known to be associated with a number of systemic, or extrapulmonary, complications, including those related to the central nervous system (febrile seizures, Guillain–Barré syndrome, meningoencephalitis), the cardiovascular system (myocardial ischaemia, congestive cardiac failure), the renal system (renal failure from myoglobinuria, exacerbations of nephrotic syndrome), the gastrointestinal system (Reye's syndrome, gastritis, parotitis), musculoskeletal complications, haematological complications and complications related to childbirth [96]. Musculoskeletal and nervous system-related complications are seen more commonly in children, with myopathy being reported in 14–48% of children with influenza (influenza B virus), and febrile seizures being seen in about 20% of hospitalised children <5 years of age with influenza [86]. Damage to the respiratory mucosa and disruptions to bacterial flora, as a consequence of influenza, can result in invasive meningococcal infections, which are observed after some epidemics [97]. Influenza is known to cause cardiovascular complications such as myocarditis and pericarditis with dyspnoea and chest pain, arrhythmias, myocardial infarction and exacerbation of congestive cardiac failure [62, 98]. Patients with uncomplicated influenza may show abnormalities on ECG. Patients who develop fulminant myocarditis with cardiogenic shock typically do so within 2 weeks of symptom onset [98]. There is also evidence to suggest that influenza virus infection is linked to an increase in the risk of vascular complications, such as ischaemia and stroke [99].

The seriousness of the presenting illness may be gauged by the severity of symptoms and the presence of underlying comorbidities. Severity scores may be used to determine the risk of death or ICU admission. However, a study investigating eight severity scoring systems, including CURB-65 (confusion, urea >7 $mmol \cdot L^{-1}$, respiratory rate $\geqslant$30 $breaths \cdot min^{-1}$, blood pressure <90 mmHg (systolic) or $\leqslant$60 mmHg (diastolic), age $\geqslant$65 years) and the Pandemic Medical Early Warning System (PMEWS), in hospitalised influenza patients concluded that none of them was an especially good predictor of ICU admission or mortality in hospital [100]. Another study comparing PMEWS, CURB-65 and Community Assessment Tools (CATs) using data from the 2009 A(H1N1) pandemic concluded that CURB-65 and

CATs were better at predicting death in adults than PMEWS, and that CATs predicted death in children and admission to critical care facilities better than both PMEWS and CURB-65 [101].

Laboratory diagnosis

While the clinical features of respiratory viruses are easily recognisable, influenza virus aetiology can only be distinguished reliably by laboratory diagnosis. Samples collected from the upper respiratory tract are used to diagnose influenza, such as nasopharyngeal swabs, and nasal or throat swabs or washes. Nasopharyngeal swabs are the most appropriate sample for detection of influenza virus, and should be collected within 3–4 days of symptom onset in adults. As children shed influenza virus for longer periods of time, diagnosis is possible for at least 1 week. Invasive specimens such as trans-tracheal lavage, bronchoalveolar lavage or lung biopsy can be collected from the lower respiratory tract, if clinically indicated. Autopsy lung tissue can be used to confirm influenza virus as the cause of death. Important factors influencing influenza virus diagnosis are the quality of the specimen and the storage and transportation conditions to the laboratory [102]. A number of diagnostic tests are available including virus isolation, direct antigen or genome detection, and the measurement of influenza virus-specific antibodies in serological assays. The sensitivity and specificity of these different tests varies according to the type of test used, the time from onset of illness to specimen collection, the type of specimen tested, the specimen quality and the laboratory performing the test. Accurate and timely influenza virus diagnosis allows early use of anti-influenza drugs, reduces inappropriate use of antibiotics and is important in infection control.

During a suspected influenza outbreak, culture of virus in cell culture or embyronated hens' eggs provides information on the circulating influenza virus strains. Culture of influenza virus strains may also provide new candidate strains of virus that can be included in the influenza vaccine for the next season through the WHO GISRS. Isolation of viruses takes at least 3 days before results are available, but allows testing of virus sensitivity to anti-influenza drugs. Virus culture is gradually being replaced in routine diagnostic practice by the more cost-effective and highly specific method of detecting the influenza virus genome in respiratory samples using RT-PCR [103]. In this assay, the viral RNA genome is transcribed by RT to DNA, which can then be amplified by PCR allowing typing (A, B or C) and subtyping for influenza A viruses according to the HA and NA. Conventional RT-PCR is being replaced by real-time RT-PCR, which allows multiplexing of a number of respiratory pathogens, with results often available on the same working day. Detection of viral antigens by immunofluorescence of clinical samples or virus isolates using influenza virus-specific monoclonal antibodies is a rapid and sensitive method for diagnosis of influenza; in addition, viral isolates can be used for HA inhibition assays. However, the assay is dependent on good-quality clinical samples, which must be processed rapidly within 1–2 h of collection. For influenza serology, paired acute ($\leqslant$7 days after symptom onset) and convalescent (2–4 weeks after disease onset) serum samples need to be collected to show an increase in antibody titre over time by a haemagglutination-inhibition or complement-fixation assay. These serological assays do not provide a rapid diagnosis and are no longer conducted routinely in virological diagnostic laboratories, but are still used in research and public health work.

NPTs provide rapid influenza virus diagnosis in 15–30 min at the point of care. In children, NPTs can reduce the need for invasive procedures such as lumbar puncture [104].

A range of NPTs is available, which can detect only influenza A virus, or both influenza A and B viruses. The type of respiratory samples collected varies with the kit, and the manufacturer's instructions should be followed carefully for each test. The majority of NPTs are immunoassays detecting NP. They have reduced sensitivities (50–70%) compared with RT-PCR or virus culture, leading to false-negative results, but high specificities (>90%) [105, 106]. During a suspected influenza outbreak, the WHO recommends confirmation of negative NPTs by RT-PCR, immunofluorescence or virus culture, alongside current influenza surveillance. Thus, a positive NPT result is useful to confirm a decision to start antiviral treatment for influenza, but a negative NPT result does not justify withholding antiviral treatment if influenza is clinically suspected.

Histopathology

In humans, influenza can occur as a range of diseases from subclinical infection to fatal fulminant pneumonia, with variable histopathological changes in proportion to severity. In uncomplicated influenza infection, the virus replicates predominantly in the upper respiratory tract, with peak viral titres detected after 2 days (correlating with fever), although virus can be detected for up to 6 days after infection. The histological changes in the respiratory tract are nonspecific and need to be supported by laboratory confirmation of influenza diagnosis detecting the viral genome or antigens. Influenza facilitates secondary bacterial infections, commonly caused by *S. pneumoniae*, *S. aureus*, *H. influenzae* or *S. pyogenes* (reviewed in [94]). In autopsy cases of severe pneumonia, typical interstitial findings are oedema and inflammatory infiltrates, the formation of hyaline membranes in the alveoli and diffuse alveolar damage, in addition to necrotising bronchitis and bronchiolitis (reviewed in [107]).

Antiviral therapy and other potential treatments

Until 1999, the adamantanes (amantadine and rimantadine) were the only antiviral drugs available for prophylaxis and treatment of influenza. These drugs inhibit M2 ion channel activity in influenza A viruses and interfere with the uncoating of influenza A virions, thereby inhibiting nuclear migration of viral RNPs and replication [108, 109]. A major limitation of these drugs has been the rapid emergence of resistance (especially when used for treatment and prophylaxis in the same setting) as a result of amino acid substitutions in the transmembrane part of the M2 protein, which either reduce binding of the M2 inhibitor or enlarge the M2 pore diameter such that its function is retained. In recent years, the S31N mutation among circulating influenza A(H3N2) and pandemic A(H1N1) influenza strains has resulted in very widespread resistance to adamantanes [110]. Other limitations include the absence of activity against influenza B virus, and frequent central nervous system side-effects (*e.g.* anxiety, hallucinations, nightmares and confusion), particularly so in elderly subjects in whom the elimination half-life may be doubled [109, 110].

From 1999 onwards, the NIs zanamivir (tradename Relenza, available as a powder for oral inhalation, and licensed for treatment and prophylaxis in patients ⩾5 years of age) and oseltamivir (tradename Tamiflu, available as oral capsules and suspension, and licensed for treatment and prophylaxis in patients of all ages) have been the most widely used antivirals for influenza treatment and prophylaxis [109, 111, 112]. NIs block the replication of both influenza A and B viruses by preventing the release of virions from the surface of infected cells [113], although one study has suggested a slightly lower effectiveness against influenza B viruses [114].

An updated Cochrane review and meta-analysis of randomised placebo-controlled trials of oseltamivir conducted between 1997 and 2004 for regulatory purposes found faster symptom relief by about 1 day and a significant reduction in self-reported pneumonia in previously healthy adults with naturally occurring influenza [115]. Subsequently, a more rigorous individual patient data meta-analysis of the same data commissioned by the European Multiparty Group for Advice on Science (MUGAS) foundation confirmed faster symptom relief (25.2 h), 44% fewer lower respiratory tract infections and 63% fewer hospitalisations associated with influenza in oseltamivir-treated adults [116]. A systematic review of observational data for both seasonal and pandemic influenza commissioned by the WHO showed that both oseltamivir and zanamivir reduced hospitalisation and the duration of symptoms [117]. Finally, an individual patient data meta-analysis of observational data on nearly 30000 hospitalised pandemic influenza patients from 78 centres found that NI use was associated with a significant 18% reduction in mortality among adults, with early administration (within 2 days of symptom onset) halving mortality. There was a decreasing effect with each day that treatment initiation was delayed; however, later treatment could still benefit critically ill patients, reducing the odds of mortality by 35% [118]. In a follow-up analysis, the authors also reported that early NI treatment significantly reduced the need for ventilator support and mortality in influenza-related pneumonia cases [119]. It is important to note that none of these studies has been able to establish a statistically significant effect of NIs with regard to more serious influenza-related outcomes in children; thus, clinical judgement should be exercised when prescribing these drugs in children. A double-blind RCT conducted in Bangladesh on influenza patients diagnosed within 5 days of symptom onset reported that oseltamivir was associated with a reduction in the duration of major symptoms by 1 day and reduced virus shedding [120], suggesting that the therapeutic window might extend beyond the licensed 2 days after symptom onset to about 5 days.

Oseltamivir has been associated with nausea and vomiting in some users, but no serious adverse effects have been reported [116]. In 2007, Japan suspended the use of oseltamivir in patients aged 10–19 years due to concerns about neuropsychiatric adverse effects including hallucinations and delirious behaviour, resulting in some self-harming incidents and fatal falls. An investigation into these concerns using Japanese vital statistics data for 10–19-year-olds from 1995 to 2005 revealed no significant increases in deaths by accident or suicide after the introduction of oseltamivir in 2001 [121]. The investigation suggested that any possible abnormal behaviour could be linked to the influenza virus infection itself, rather than to oseltamivir. Major public health authorities recommend the use of NIs in patients at increased risk of influenza complications or who are seriously unwell with influenza [122–124].

Surveillance data on seasonal influenza virus strains show that resistance to all NIs is currently low (~2%), and NIs remain an appropriate choice for influenza treatment and prophylaxis [125]. Resistant strains have been seen more commonly in oseltamivir-treated children infected with pre-pandemic A(H1N1) viruses (>99%) with low resistance to A(H3N2) and the pandemic strain A(H1N1)pdm09 (<3%), and almost no resistance has been observed among A(H5N1) viruses [126]. The first reports of widespread resistance to oseltamivir in Europe emerged in 2007–2008, when about 14% of seasonal (pre-pandemic) influenza A(H1N1) viruses in surveillance specimens carried the H275Y neuraminidase mutation associated with oseltamivir resistance [127, 128], although in some localities this was almost 70% [129]; however, this did not seem to be linked to oseltamivir use [130, 131]. By the end of 2008, oseltamivir-resistant A(H1N1) had completely displaced oseltamivir-sensitive A(H1N1) viruses across the globe, until displaced by the oseltamivir-sensitive A(H1N1)pdm09 pandemic virus in 2009, which remains in seasonal circulation [132]. A slow clinical response, or relapse of symptoms, or a slow virological response as evidenced by quantitative PCR should alert clinicians to the possibility of resistance. Increasing the dosage of oseltamivir has not been shown to benefit patients infected with H275Y-mediated oseltamivir-resistant strains; however, most cases remain susceptible to zanamivir, and other therapeutic options might include ribavirin or laninamivir [133, 134]. *In vivo* animal models and mathematical modelling of human infection have suggested that triple-combination antiviral therapy comprising adamantanes, NIs and possibly ribavirin would act synergistically against drug-resistant influenza viruses [110, 135, 136]. Perelson *et al.* [136] recommended using such drug combinations in immunocompromised and severely ill viral pneumonia patients.

Other NIs include peramivir (licensed for use in Japan as Rapiacta, in South Korea as Peramiflu and more recently by the US Food and Drug Administration (FDA) in 2014 as an intravenous administration of a single dose of 600 mg in adults ⩾18 years of age under the tradename Rapivab) [137]. Clinical trial data show that a single intravenous dose of peramivir may be an alternative to a 5-day oral dose of oseltamivir in patients unable to tolerate an oral dose, as well as improving compliance and providing stable pharmacokinetics in other patients with uncomplicated influenza [138, 139]. Diarrhoea, nausea and vomiting are the commonly reported adverse effects, although a phase III trial found no significant difference in adverse effects experienced due to peramivir and oseltamivir [138, 140]. Laninamivir (tradename Inavir) was approved for influenza treatment in Japan in 2010 and for prophylaxis in 2013, and is available as a long-acting NI administered in a single dose by nasal inhalation. It has performed well in *in vitro* studies against wild-type influenza A and B viruses and has been shown to inhibit neuraminidase activity in oseltamivir-resistant viruses [110, 141]. In clinical studies, laninamivir has demonstrated noninferiority *versus* oseltamivir, and common adverse effects include diarrhoea, nausea, vomiting and dizziness [110].

Other antiviral agents currently being evaluated for influenza treatment and prophylaxis in clinical trials include favipiravir (T-705), nitazoxanide and Fludase (DAS181) [142]. Fludase has shown antiviral activity against a range of influenza A and B viruses *in vitro* and in animal models [143]. Fludase removes SA-containing receptors from respiratory epithelial cells, preventing the attachment and replication of influenza virus [143]. In a placebo-controlled phase II study in patients with uncomplicated influenza, Fludase significantly reduced viral load and the duration of virus shedding [144]. Favipiravir selectively inhibits the RNA-dependent RNA polymerase of influenza viruses, directly inhibiting virus replication and transcription, and has demonstrated *in vitro* activity against a range of RNA viruses including filoviruses, flaviviruses, bunyaviruses, arenaviruses, noroviruses, influenza A viruses (H1N1, H2N2 and H3N2), and influenza B and C viruses; moreover, viruses resistant to both oseltamivir and zanamivir were susceptible to favipiravir [145, 146]. *In vivo* studies of favipiravir in mice have demonstrated protection against lethal infection by a variety of influenza strains with similar or greater inhibitory activity than oseltamivir and zanamivir against some strains. Phase II/III trials in humans have established a good safety profile for favipiravir; however, because of previously demonstrated links to teratogenicity (including external, internal and skeletal anomalies) in animal studies, the drug has so far obtained limited licensure in Japan, restricting its use to during outbreaks of antiviral medication-resistant influenza [147, 148]. Nitazoxanide, originally developed as an antiprotozoal agent, has been repurposed as a broad-spectrum antiviral drug with good activity *in vitro* against influenza A viruses, demonstrating low resistance and synergistic activity with oseltamivir or zanamivir [149]. It acts by blocking the maturation of viral HA at the post-translational level, thereby inhibiting virus replication [150]. A phase IIb/III placebo-controlled clinical trial of nitazoxanide (600 mg twice daily for 5 days) in uncomplicated influenza cases found a significant reduction in time to alleviation of symptoms (median duration of symptoms 95.5 h (95% CI 84.0–108.0 h) compared with 116.7 h (95% CI 108.1–122.1 h) in the placebo group) with activity against both influenza A and B viruses, and no significant difference in adverse events between the treatment and placebo groups [150].

In addition to antiviral agents, anti-inflammatory drugs can be used to modulate the innate immune response to influenza viruses. Corticosteroids are already widely used for the treatment of severe influenza on the premise that they can reduce acute inflammation, but concerns have been expressed about unintended detrimental effects because of increased virus replication, given the immunosuppressive effects of these drugs [151]. These concerns have now been validated by two recent systematic reviews of observational studies and an individual patient data meta-analysis of three Asian surveillance cohorts, which found that systematic corticosteroid therapy for presumed influenza-associated complications was associated with a significant increase in mortality, nosocomial infection, and the duration of mechanical ventilation and ICU stay [152–154]. Rodrigo *et al.* [153] recommended that systemic corticosteroid therapy should not be used in influenza infections unless indicated for other reasons, such as vasopressor-dependent septic shock. In recent years, there have also been a number of observational studies supporting the potential immunomodulatory effects of statins in a range of infections [155]. These effects are biologically plausible, given the demonstration *in vitro* that statins affect several cellular pathways that can inhibit influenza virus proliferation [156]. However, *in vivo* data in mice are inconclusive [155], and in the absence of clinical trials, the use of these drugs for influenza patients should be deferred to clinical judgement in individual cases.

In severe influenza infections, it may be worthwhile considering immunotherapy with convalescent plasma and intravenous immunoglobulin. Convalescent serum contains neutralising antibodies, which may aid recovery in severely ill patients *via* passive immunity. A recent systematic review found that convalescent plasma for the treatment of SARIs of viral aetiology may reduce mortality by at least 55%, especially if administered early after symptom onset, and did not find evidence of serious adverse events [157]. However, the authors acknowledged the low quality of the available data. Other studies have investigated the use of anti-influenza virus hyperimmune intravenous immunoglobulin (hIVIg) prepared from pooled plasma from convalescent patients or from healthy volunteers recently vaccinated against either seasonal or pandemic strains of influenza viruses. A recent pilot study of adults with seasonal influenza demonstrated that administration of hIVIg could result in a strain-specific HA antibody response that occurred at least 3 days earlier than with natural infection, and a clinical effectiveness trial is underway (ClinicalTrials.gov identifier: NCT02008578) [158]. There is also growing interest in identifying and engineering synthetic antibodies that could neutralise influenza virus. Promising candidates include broadly neutralising antibodies that bind to the various subtypes of influenza HA; *in vitro* and *in vivo* tests have demonstrated the ability of these antibodies to protect against multiple strains of influenza, with the theoretical possibility of reducing secondary bacterial infection due to the reduction in viral titres, which prevents bacterial adherence [159]. It is important to note, however, that resistance can also develop to antibodies due to antigenic drift and shift; therefore, an effective immunotherapy should aim to target an epitope that is considered stable.

Since the 2009 pandemic, there has been increased use of extracorporeal membrane oxygenation (ECMO) to deliver cardiorespiratory support in patients with refractory hypoxaemia secondary to severe influenza pneumonia complicated by ARDS. Studies of

ECMO for the treatment of severe influenza are limited to observational data from the 2009 A(H1N1)pdm09 pandemic, but overall do not clearly indicate a beneficial effect compared with standard ICU care [160–162].

Study designs and end-points for monitoring antiviral therapy

The FDA guidance for industry [163] on the evaluation of influenza antivirals approves the use of placebo-controlled trials in patients with acute uncomplicated influenza, as the risk to trial participants from nontreatment is expected to be small. In addition, superiority trials with approved antivirals are recommended. However, in the case of more serious influenza requiring hospitalisation, the FDA recommends a superiority add-on trial, in which a combination of the investigational drug and approved (standard of care) therapy is shown to be superior to the standard of care when used alone. Recommended primary efficacy end-points for uncomplicated influenza include the duration of influenza symptoms using patient-reported measures with secondary virological end-points such as viral load. Other secondary clinical end-points include the time to return to normal activity and the time to resolution of fever, with emergence of drug resistance being a tertiary end-point. For seriously ill, hospitalised patients, primary end-points include clinical signs and symptoms, the duration of hospitalisation, the time to normalisation of vital signs and oxygenation, the requirements for supplemental oxygen or mechanical ventilation, and mortality [163]. However, Ison *et al.* [164] advocated the use of virological measures, such as replication, as primary end-points in severely ill, hospitalised patients, the rationale being that comorbidities and other host factors may influence ultimate clinical outcomes, and thus evidence of influenza virus clearance may serve as a more objective marker of antiviral efficacy.

The regulatory evidence for the commonly used NI antivirals, notably oseltamivir, comes from clinical trials of previously healthy subjects with uncomplicated influenza, which show marginal benefits, such as faster resolution of symptoms by about a day [115]. This evidence has limited generalizability to severe influenza cases, and the ethical considerations around withholding potentially beneficial antiviral treatment from more severely ill patients make the conduct of placebo-controlled clinical trials in such settings difficult or even impossible. Moreover, even for superiority trials, it is much more challenging to recruit sufficient numbers of patients to ensure that the trials are adequately powered to detect significant improvements with regard to rare outcomes such as influenza-related mortality. Therefore, the best evidence to date with regard to mortality and influenza-related complications such as pneumonia and the need for secondary or critical care comes from observational studies. While observational data are vulnerable to bias and confounding by treatment indication, advances in statistical methods, such as propensity scoring, can overcome these limitations to a reasonable extent, allowing valid causal inferences regarding antiviral effectiveness [165].

Vaccines

Types of influenza vaccines

The first influenza vaccines were introduced in 1945 and were inactivated influenza vaccines (IIVs) [166]. Early vaccines were whole-virus inactivated vaccines consisting of crudely purified whole virus inactivated with formalin and phenylmercuric nitrate. Present-day IIVs include various formulations of chemically inactivated influenza virus such as whole virus, split virion (where the virus is split using ether and/or detergent), subunit (where the influenza virus surface proteins, HA and NA, are purified and enriched) or virosomal [167, 168]. Virosomes are lipid-based virus-like particles consisting of reconstituted influenza virus envelopes without the viral genetic material [167]. In addition, IIVs are available in adjuvanted and nonadjuvanted formulations. Adjuvants increase the immunogenicity of highly purified antigens that have inadequate immunostimulatory properties. The most commonly used seasonal influenza vaccine adjuvant is MF59, with AS03 used in the recent pandemic influenza vaccine; both are oil-in-water adjuvant emulsions containing squalene (a fully metabolisable oil source from shark liver oil) and enhance the innate immune response involved in the recognition of pathogen-associated molecular patterns on the basis of which foreign matter is classified as a threat [169]. Moreover, adjuvants have an antigen dose-sparing function, as less viral antigen is required per dose, and thus global vaccine production capacity may be increased during a pandemic [170].

Live attenuated influenza viruses (LAIVs) utilise a single attenuated vaccine virus or master donor viruses (MDVs) containing a mutation for attenuation. There are MDVs for both influenza A and B viruses (A/Ann Arbor/6/60 H2N2 and B/Ann Arbor/1/66) containing a number of mutations in the internal genes that render them temperature sensitive, cold adapted and attenuated. Novel attenuated influenza viruses representing the circulating virus strains were produced initially by reassortment with the MDV, using the time-consuming classical reassortment technique involving simultaneous co-infection of embryonated chicken eggs with the wild-type strain and MDV, followed by repeated passaging in embryonated eggs. Newer influenza vaccine methods involve the use of a synthetic virus seed produced *via* reverse genetics, but may be subject to intellectual property rights and regulations on genetically modified organisms [171]. LAIVs have been recommended for children due to the low immunogenicity of IIVs in this group [170] and the ease of administration. Influenza vaccines are manufactured primarily *via* virus culture in embryonated hens' eggs, and less frequently *via* cell culture [166]. IIVs can be administered *via* either intramuscular or intradermal routes, while current LAIVs are administered intranasally. LAIVs are associated with better immunogenicity than IIVs, particularly in children, but lower tolerability [169], and existing guidelines contraindicate their use in severely immunocompromised individuals, individuals with severe asthma, and children and adolescents receiving salicylate therapy (because of concerns about Reye's syndrome with salicylates and wild-type influenza infection) [172, 173]. However, a recent multicentre prospective cohort study of the safety of LAIVs in young people (2–18 years of age) found that the vaccine was well tolerated in those with asthma or recurring wheeze; in addition, it found a low risk of systemic allergic reactions in young people with egg allergy [174]. Intradermal vaccines are dose sparing, as they require 40% less antigen (the human dermis and epidermis are rich in antigen-presenting cells) than intramuscular vaccines and require a much smaller needle diameter, making them more amenable to individuals who dislike needles. There is no evidence of a significant difference in immunological response when comparing intradermal and intramuscular influenza vaccines in the general population; however, higher doses of intradermal vaccines produced a better immune response in older adults >60 years of age [175, 176].

Seasonal influenza vaccines are prepared using virus strains recommended by the WHO each year (in February for the northern hemisphere and in September for the southern hemisphere) [172]. Vaccine mismatch with circulating virus strains can occur, for example, during the 2014–2015 influenza season, resulting in reduced vaccine effectiveness, but this is infrequent [173, 177]. Most current inactivated influenza vaccines are trivalent, containing two subtypes of influenza A virus and one influenza B virus; more recently, quadrivalent vaccines with viruses from both influenza B virus lineages have been developed [173]. Quadrivalent vaccines are considered an improvement over trivalent vaccines, as the inclusion of a second influenza B virus lineage diminishes the probability of a vaccine mismatch [173], which occurs relatively frequently [178]. LAIVs provide broader protection than inactivated vaccines and could offer better protection against strains that have undergone antigenic drift leading to a vaccine mismatch [179]. High-dose influenza vaccines have been recommended in people ⩾65 years of age because of lower immunogenicity with age. DiazGranados *et al.* [180] reported that a high-dose trivalent IIV containing four times as much HA as standard-dose vaccines was 24.2% more effective in preventing influenza in adults ⩾65 years of age compared with the standard-dose vaccine. The safety profile of the high-dose vaccine was similar to that of the standard-dose vaccine, and no vaccine-related serious adverse events were identified by the investigators [180].

Vaccine production approaches

Although most influenza vaccine manufacturing platforms still involve virus propagation in fertilised hens' eggs, there are significant disadvantages to this approach, including challenges around procuring sufficient vaccine-quality eggs to meet the global vaccine demand, and the need for egg-adapted reassortment strains that will grow efficiently in eggs. The latter requirement increases the likelihood of mutations in the reassorted virus that could contribute further to a vaccine mismatch [181]. An alternative to this is cell culture-based manufacturing approaches in which the wild-type virus can be grown directly in a cell-line and then used in either whole-virus vaccines (either LAIVs or IIVs after being inactivated), or is separated into constituent proteins for use in split-virus or subunit-type vaccines. Theoretically, cell-based approaches are more conducive to large scale-up, but only a few cell-based manufacturing facilities are currently approved, because of the large investment required to set up and quality control these facilities and adapt wild-type influenza strains for cell culture. Madin–Darby canine kidney cells were the first cells used for seasonal influenza vaccine manufacture using cell culture-based approaches; other cell lines include Vero (monkey kidney cells; licensed for pre-pandemic IIV and split-virion vaccines in the European Union and Japan), human retina-derived PER.C6, human embryonic kidney (HEK-293) and amniocyte-derived cell lines (the latter two are still in pre-clinical development) [182]. Another advantage of cell-based vaccine manufacturing approaches is increased vaccine purity. An alternative manufacturing approach is the use of baculovirus expression vector systems in which the baculovirus vector, rather than the full virus, is used for the rapid production of the HA antigen in insect cells. This approach is used for the production of recombinant influenza subunit vaccines and has the advantages of being able to skip inactivation and purification steps, and producing a more predictable yield of antigen [182]. Yet another alternative to animal cell-culture approaches is using plant-based expression of the HA antigen. This can be done by a number of methods: the incorporation of transgenes into the nuclear or chloroplast genome of plants (stable transformant strategies) or by developing transient expression systems including the infiltration of plants with *Agrobacterium* carrying a binary vector, infection of plants with a modified plant virus, or a combination of viral vector-based or *Agrobacterium*-mediated methods. Transient expression systems offer faster production cycles than stable transformant systems. The most commonly used plant genus for plant-based expression approaches is *Nicotiana* (the tobacco plant family) or its hybrids [183]. Soema *et al.* [181] have provided a detailed review of current and novel vaccine manufacturing approaches.

Evidence for influenza vaccine effectiveness

Vaccine efficacy (V_E) can be measured using both clinical (laboratory-confirmed and syndromic case definitions of influenza) and serological end-points; however, the latter can overestimate V_E, as it is difficult to differentiate post-vaccination increases in antibody titres from post-infection increases, and therefore using RT-PCR for virus identification is recommended [184]. Kavanagh *et al.* [185] demonstrated that V_E estimates varied, depending on the outcome measure and methodological approach used. Using the same dataset, they showed that the effectiveness of the pandemic vaccine was between 34% and 60% using different methodological approaches, with the best V_E estimates obtained for the virology-confirmed subset of symptomatic individuals [185].

A systematic Cochrane review of RCTs concluded that IIVs were modestly effective in preventing ILI and laboratory-confirmed influenza in healthy adults based on a pooled V_E of 16% against ILI, which increased to 60% for confirmed influenza and 62% when the vaccine matched the circulating virus strain [186]. LAIVs had an overall V_E against confirmed influenza of 53%. The review found no significant association between influenza vaccination and adverse effects. Another Cochrane review including both RCTs and observational studies found that LAIVs were 80% effective in preventing laboratory-confirmed influenza in healthy children [115]. In a third Cochrane review, in people with asthma, no significant reduction in influenza-related asthma exacerbations was found between the vaccinated and placebo groups [187]. All the above reviews acknowledged the relatively low quality of RCTs included in their analysis, as well as the heterogeneity of methods used.

In 2008, the European Centre for Disease Prevention and Control (ECDC) established the Influenza Monitoring Vaccine Effectiveness (I-MOVE) network to monitor seasonal and pandemic influenza vaccine effectiveness in Europe in a standardised way. The I-MOVE network uses robust case definitions involving virological confirmation of influenza and methodological approaches that minimise selection bias and confounding [188]. Table 2 summarises V_E estimates from the I-MOVE network from 2008/2009 to 2013/2014, illustrating the importance of a good vaccine match with circulating viruses.

In addition, continued surveillance of influenza V_E across the globe shows consistent benefits from seasonal influenza vaccination in adults, children and high-risk groups, ranging from 20% to as high as 70% when there is a good vaccine match with circulating virus strains [166]. Moreover, using a less stratified approach, it is possible to demonstrate significant benefits from influenza vaccination, even in the elderly, in contrast to the conclusions of a Cochrane review (V_E against ILI of ~40%, V_E against disease with confirmed virus infection of ~50% and biological vaccine efficacy when there is a vaccine match of ~60%) [195]. Finally, a meta-analysis by Beck *et al.* [196] found that influenza vaccination offered significant protection against both ILI and confirmed influenza in immunocompromised patients.

Recommendations for seasonal influenza vaccination

Seasonal influenza vaccination has been recommended by the ECDC for patients at high risk of influenza infection and its complications; this includes patients with chronic diseases, such as COPD, asthma, congestive heart disease, chronic heart failure, diabetes, chronic renal disease,

Table 2. Influenza vaccine efficacy estimates from the Influenza Monitoring Vaccine Effectiveness network (2008/2009 to 2013/2014 influenza seasons)

First author [ref.]	Countries covered	Subjects	Influenza season	Vaccine type and match with circulating strain	Vaccine effectiveness % (95% CI)
Kissling [189]	Denmark, Hungary, Portugal, Romania, Spain	138 cases and 189 test-negative controls; ⩾65 years of age.	2008–2009	Trivalent inactivated influenza vaccine; vaccine match for A strain; mismatch for B strain.	Crude: 55.1 (27.8–72.1); adjusted[#]: 59.1 (15.3–80.3); adjusted[#] against A(H3) strain (vaccine match): 56.4 (0.2–81.0).
Valenciano [188]	France, Hungary, Ireland, Italy, Romania, Portugal, Spain	918 cases and 1984 test-negative controls; all ages.	2009–2010	Pandemic influenza vaccine; vaccine matched to pandemic A(H1N1)pdm09 strain.	Crude: 79.0 (55.8–90.0); adjusted[¶]: 66.0 (23.9–84.8).
Kissling [190]	France, Hungary, Ireland, Italy, Romania, Portugal, Spain, Poland	2019 cases and 2391 test-negative controls; all ages.	2010–2011	Trivalent inactivated influenza vaccine (adjuvanted and non-adjuvanted); good match for circulating A and B strains.	Crude: 65.5 (53.2–74.6); adjusted[+]: 50.9 (25.2–67.7).
Kissling [191, 192]	Romania, Hungary, Ireland, Italy, Poland, Portugal, Spain, France	Early season estimates: 206 cases and 327 test-negative controls; all ages. Overall season estimates: 440 cases and 581 test-negative controls; all ages.	2011–2012	Seasonal vaccine type not specified; limited match with circulating A(H3) strain.	Early season estimates: crude: 42.9 (10.3–63.6); adjusted[§]: 43.0 (−0.4–67.7). Overall season estimates: crude: 12.2 (−17.2–34.2); adjusted[§]: 24.8 (−5.6–46.5).
Kissling [193]	Romania, Hungary, Ireland, Italy, Poland, Portugal, Spain, France	3653 cases and 2772 test-negative controls; all ages.	2012–2013	Trivalent inactivated influenza vaccine (adjuvanted and nonadjuvanted; subunit and split virion); three influenza types/subtypes in circulation.	Crude (influenza B virus): 46.5 (30.9–58.6); adjusted[f] (influenza B virus): 49.3 (32.4–62.0). Crude (influenza A/H1N1 pdm09): 56.1 (38.6–68.7); adjusted[f] (influenza A/H1N1 pdm09): 50.4 (28.4–65.6). Crude (influenza A/H3N2): 22.5 (−8.6–44.7); adjusted[f] (influenza A/H3N2): 42.2 (14.9–60.7).

Continued

Table 2. Continued

First author [ref.]	Countries covered	Subjects	Influenza season	Vaccine type and match with circulating strain	Vaccine effectiveness % (95% CI)
Valenciano [194]	Germany, Hungary, Ireland, Portugal, Romania and Spain	A(H1N1)pdm09 analysis: 531 cases and 1712 test-negative controls; all ages. A(H3N2) analysis: 623 cases and 1920 test-negative controls; all ages.	2013–2014	Trivalent inactivated influenza vaccine (subunit, split virion, adjuvanted); circulating viruses antigenically similar to vaccine virus but some heterogeneity in circulating viruses by study site and amino acid mutations in the B antigenic site.	Crude (influenza A/H1N1 pdm09): 52.2 (30.3–67.3); adjusted[##] (influenza A/H1N1 pdm09): 47.5 (16.4–67.0); adjusted[##] (A/H3N2): 30.2 (−33.9–63.6); 51.5% heterogeneity between study sites: adjusted[##] (A/H3N2) for sites, range 3.6–90.2%.

[#]: adjusted for study centre, age, sex, presence of chronic conditions, previous hospitalisations, smoking history, functional status and previous influenza vaccination; [¶]: adjusted for 2009–2010 seasonal influenza vaccine, influenza vaccine in the previous two seasons, presence of chronic conditions, sex, age, hospitalisation in previous year, smoking history, visits to general practitioner in previous year and month of symptom onset; [+]: adjusted for age, sex, presence of chronic conditions, hospitalisations in previous year, smoking status, visits to general practitioner in previous year, 2009–2010 pandemic vaccination status, seasonal influenza vaccination 2009–2010 and week of symptom onset; [§]: adjusted for age, sex, presence of chronic conditions, hospitalisations in previous year, visits to general practitioner in previous year and week of symptom onset; [f]: adjusted for onset week, chronic condition, age and sex; [##]: adjusted for study site, onset week, age, chronic conditions and sex.

chronic liver disease, stroke, asplenia or splenic dysfunction, and immunocompromised patients [197–199]. Seasonal influenza vaccination has also been recommended for the elderly (⩾65 years of age) and pregnant women [173, 197, 200]. In the UK, seasonal influenza vaccination was introduced for all healthy children aged 2–17 years in September 2013 [173]. There is already evidence that this new programme has reduced the overall illness burden in children and adults [201, 202]. The Centers for Disease Control and Prevention (CDC), on the other hand, goes further by recommending annual influenza vaccination for all individuals of ⩾6 months of age, unless there is a contraindication [172]. Recent US data suggest that this approach is cost-effective and sometimes even cost-saving [203]. In addition, seasonal influenza vaccination has been recommended for health and social care professionals who may come into contact with patients, to reduce the transmission of influenza virus and protect those with suboptimal immunogenicity to vaccines [173].

Controversies

Influenza virus vaccines are generally well tolerated as outlined above; however, a number of controversies related to potential adverse effects have affected influenza vaccination uptake. HABER *et al.* [204] reported an unexplained increase in the risk of Guillain–Barré syndrome in recipients of the swine influenza vaccine in 1976; other studies have found no association between Guillain–Barré syndrome and influenza vaccination, although a strong association has been found with ILI [173, 205]. Newer data suggested a small increased risk of Guillain–Barré syndrome following the 2009 pandemic influenza vaccine (one to three additional cases per million vaccinees), but, given the lack of conclusive evidence due to potential confounding, the benefits of influenza vaccination need to be weighed against this possible increased risk by policy makers, clinicians and potential vaccine recipients [206]. Similarly, an increased risk of narcolepsy was identified after vaccination with the AS03-adjuvanted pandemic A(H1N1) 2009 vaccine Pandemrix [207, 208]. While it has not been possible to attribute causation [209], there is nevertheless a theoretical possibility that adjuvants used in vaccine formulations may induce unwanted immune reactions, and active surveillance of vaccine-associated adverse events is therefore of paramount importance [169].

Advances in universal influenza vaccine development

The need to continually update the annual seasonal influenza vaccine because of antigenic drift, concerns around vaccine mismatch and the late arrival of pandemic vaccines in 2009 have sustained efforts to develop a universal influenza vaccine that could afford protection against all influenza virus strains. The key concept for universal influenza vaccine development is the identification of conserved epitopes that exist across influenza virus subtypes [210]. Promising epitopes include the stalk region of the HA glycoprotein (either with the head removed or with a different head, resulting in a chimeric HA), the extracellular component of the influenza A virus M2 protein, which is a transmembrane protein involved in virus uncoating, the globular head of the NA surface protein (as NA antigenic drift rates are generally lower than those for the globular head of the HA) and T-cell-activating influenza A virus NP and M1 [168, 181]. One of the challenges of focusing on conserved epitopes is their relatively poor immunogenicity, which is why simultaneous development of better adjuvants and vaccine delivery platforms (*e.g.* virus vectors, which are genetically modified viruses and nanoparticles) is required [211]. Significant uncertainties remain about the timescales for development of a universal influenza vaccine and its eventual breadth and duration of protection; both will need to be considerable in order for this to be a viable replacement for annual vaccination by IIVs and LAIVs.

Conclusion

Interpandemic influenza imposes a large public health burden, with two subtypes of influenza A virus and two distinct lineages of influenza B virus in constant global circulation. Antigenic drift is responsible for recurrent outbreaks and epidemics, and explains why influenza vaccine composition requires annual review and frequent updating. In temperate zones, influenza virus activity is highly seasonal, but less so in tropical and equatorial regions. Most cases of influenza occur in children, and overall at least 50% of cases are asymptomatic. Nevertheless, interpandemic influenza is consistently associated with excess population mortality during epidemics, with the burden of severe or complicated illness usually centred on children <6 months of age, the elderly, persons with underlying chronic conditions, pregnant women and the morbidly obese. In patients with mild influenza, NIs reduce the duration of symptoms by about 1 day, with a possible reduction in hospitalisation, but in adults hospitalised with influenza, NIs have a clearer effect in reducing mortality, especially if commenced early. Currently, resistance to NIs is low, but this has the potential to change rapidly. There is now clear evidence that corticosteroids given to severely unwell patients with influenza adversely affect mortality, nosocomial infections and the duration of ventilation. Influenza vaccines are the established means of primary prevention, with live attenuated vaccines preferred to inactivated vaccines in children, and quadrivalent vaccines reducing the chances of influenza B virus mismatch. Although individual clinical effectiveness is modest, the public health rationale for vaccination of at-risk patients is well established. Nevertheless, improved vaccines are needed that offer increased, broader and more enduring protection.

References

1. Simonsen L, Clarke MJ, Schonberger LB, *et al.* Pandemic versus epidemic influenza mortality: a pattern of changing age distribution. *J Infect Dis* 1998; 178: 53–60.
2. van den Wijngaard CC, van Asten L, Koopmans MPG, *et al.* Comparing pandemic to seasonal influenza mortality: moderate impact overall but high mortality in young children. *PLoS One* 2012; 7: e31197.
3. Nair H, Brooks WA, Katz M, *et al.* Global burden of respiratory infections due to seasonal influenza in young children: a systematic review and meta-analysis. *Lancet* 2011; 378: 1917–1930.
4. Poehling KA, Edwards KM, Weinberg GA, *et al.* The underrecognized burden of influenza in young children. *N Engl J Med* 2006; 355: 31–40.
5. Hause BM, Collin EA, Liu R, *et al.* Characterization of a novel influenza virus in cattle and swine: proposal for a new genus in the *Orthomyxoviridae* family. *MBio* 2014; 5: e00031-14.
6. Rota PA, Wallis TR, Harmon MW, *et al.* Cocirculation of two distinct evolutionary lineages of influenza type B virus since 1983. *Virology* 1990; 175: 59–68.
7. Fonville J, Wilks S, James S, *et al.* Antibody landscapes after influenza virus infection or vaccination. *Science* 2014; 346: 996–1000.
8. Garten RJ, Davis CT, Russell CA, *et al.* Antigenic and genetic characteristics of swine-origin 2009 A(H1N1) influenza viruses circulating in humans. *Science* 2009; 325: 197–201.
9. Biere B, Bauer B, Schweiger B. Differentiation of influenza B virus lineages Yamagata and Victoria by real-time PCR. *J Clin Microbiol* 2010; 48: 1425–1427.
10. Hay AJ, Gregory V, Douglas AR, *et al.* The evolution of human influenza viruses. *Philos Trans R Soc Lond B Biol Sci* 2001; 356: 1861–1870.
11. Kanegae Y, Sugita S, Endo A, *et al.* Evolutionary pattern of the hemagglutinin gene of influenza B viruses isolated in Japan: cocirculating lineages in the same epidemic season. *J Virol* 1990; 64: 2860–2865.
12. WHO. A Revision of the System of Nomenclature for Influenza Viruses: a WHO Memorandum. *Bull World Health Organ* 1980; 58: 585–591.

13. WHO/OIE/FAO H5N1 Evolution Working Group. Continued Evolution of Highly Pathogenic Avian Influenza A (H5N1): Updated Nomenclature. *Influenza Other Respir Viruses* 2012; 6: 1–5.
14. Wise HM, Foeglein A, Sun J, *et al.* A complicated message: identification of a novel PB1-related protein translated from influenza A virus segment 2 mRNA. *J Virol* 2009; 83: 8021–8031.
15. Muramoto Y, Noda T, Kawakami E, *et al.* Identification of novel influenza A virus proteins translated from PA mRNA. *J Virol* 2013; 87: 2455–2462.
16. Wise HM, Hutchinson EC, Jagger BW, *et al.* Identification of a novel splice variant form of the influenza A virus M2 ion channel with an antigenically distinct ectodomain. *PLoS Pathog* 2012; 8: e1002998.
17. Shaw ML, Palese P. *Orthomyxoviridae*. *In*: Knipe DM, Howley PM, eds. Fields Virology. 6th Edn. Philadelphia, Wolters Kluwer/Lippincott Williams & Wilkins Health, 2013; pp. 1151–1185.
18. Cox RJ, Brokstad KA, Ogra P. Influenza virus: immunity and vaccination strategies. Comparison of the immune response to inactivated and live, attenuated influenza vaccines. *Scand J Immunol* 2004; 59: 1–15.
19. Ye Q, Krug RM, Tao YJ. The mechanism by which influenza A virus nucleoprotein forms oligomers and binds RNA. *Nature* 2006; 444: 1078–1082.
20. Roberts KL, Manicassamy B, Lamb RA. Influenza A virus uses intercellular connections to spread to neighboring cells. *J Virol* 2015; 89: 1537–1549.
21. Skehel JJ, Wiley DC. Receptor binding and membrane fusion in virus entry: the influenza hemagglutinin. *Annu Rev Biochem* 2000; 69: 531–569.
22. de Graaf M, Fouchier RA. Role of receptor binding specificity in influenza A virus transmission and pathogenesis. *EMBO J* 2014; 33: 823–841.
23. Lakdawala SS, Jayaraman A, Halpin RA, *et al.* The soft palate is an important site of adaptation for transmissible influenza viruses. *Nature* 2015; 526: 122–125.
24. Ma W, Kahn RE, Richt JA. The pig as a mixing vessel for influenza viruses: human and veterinary implications. *J Mol Genet Med* 2009; 3: 158–166.
25. Gregory V, Bennett M, Orkhan M, *et al.* Emergence of influenza A H1N2 reassortant viruses in the human population during 2001. *Virology* 2002; 300: 1–7.
26. Finkelman BS, Viboud C, Koelle K, *et al.* Global patterns in seasonal activity of influenza A/H3N2, A/H1N1, and B from 1997 to 2005: viral coexistence and latitudinal gradients. *PLoS One* 2007; 2: e1296.
27. Hope-Simpson RE. The role of season in the epidemiology of influenza. *Epidemiol Infect* 1981; 86: 35–47.
28. Monto AS, Koopman JS, Longini IM. Tecumseh study of illness. XIII. Influenza infection and disease, 1976–1981. *Am J Epidemiol* 1985; 121: 811–822.
29. Thacker SB. The persistence of influenza A in human populations. *Epidemiol Rev* 1986; 8: 129–142.
30. Davey ML, Reid D. Relationship of air temperature to outbreaks of influenza. *Br J Prev Soc Med* 1972; 26: 28–32.
31. Jordan WS Jr. The mechanism of spread of Asian influenza 1. *Am Rev Respir Dis* 1961; 83: 29–40.
32. Fine PEM, Clarkson JA. Measles in England and Wales – I: An analysis of factors underlying seasonal patterns. *Int J Epidemiol* 1982; 11: 5–14.
33. Harper GJ. Airborne micro-organisms: survival tests with four viruses. *Epidemiol Infect* 1961; 59: 479–486.
34. Hemmes JH, Winkler KC, Kool SM. Virus survival as a seasonal factor in influenza and poliomyelitis. *Nature* 1960; 188: 430–431.
35. Schaffer F, Soergel M, Straube D. Survival of airborne influenza virus: effects of propagating host, relative humidity, and composition of spray fluids. *Arch Virol* 1976; 51: 263–273.
36. McDevitt J, Rudnick S, First M, *et al.* Role of absolute humidity in the inactivation of influenza viruses on stainless steel surfaces at elevated temperatures. *Appl Environ Microbiol* 2010; 76: 3943–3947.
37. Polozov IV, Bezrukov L, Gawrisch K, *et al.* Progressive ordering with decreasing temperature of the phospholipids of influenza virus. *Nat Chem Biol* 2008; 4: 248–255.
38. Gustin KM, Belser JA, Veguilla V, *et al.* Environmental conditions affect exhalation of H3N2 seasonal and variant influenza viruses and respiratory droplet transmission in ferrets. *PLoS One* 2015; 10: e0125874.
39. Lowen A, Palese P. Transmission of influenza virus in temperate zones is predominantly by aerosol, in the tropics by contact: A hypothesis. *PLoS Curr* 2009; 1: RRN1002.
40. Lowen AC, Mubareka S, Steel J, *et al.* Influenza virus transmission is dependent on relative humidity and temperature. *PLoS Pathog* 2007; 3: e151.
41. Brustad M, Edvardsen K, Wilsgaard T, *et al.* Seasonality of UV-radiation and vitamin D status at 69 degrees north. *Photochem Photobiol Sci* 2007; 6: 903–908.
42. Webb AR, Kline L, Holick MF. Influence of season and latitude on the cutaneous synthesis of vitamin D3: exposure to winter sunlight in Boston and Edmonton will not promote vitamin D3 synthesis in human skin. *J Clin Endocrinol Metab* 1988; 67: 373–378.
43. Urashima M, Segawa T, Okazaki M, *et al.* Randomized trial of vitamin D supplementation to prevent seasonal influenza A in schoolchildren. *Am J Clin Nutr* 2010; 91: 1255–1260.
44. Li-Ng M, Aloia jF, Pollack S, *et al.* A randomized controlled trial of vitamin D3 supplementation for the prevention of symptomatic upper respiratory tract infections. *Epidemiol Infect* 2009; 137: 1396–1404.

45. Tamerius J, Nelson MI, Zhou SZ, *et al.* Global influenza seasonality: reconciling patterns across temperate and tropical regions. *Environ Health Perspect* 2011; 119: 439.
46. Lipsitch M, Viboud C. Influenza seasonality: lifting the fog. *Proc Natl Acad Sci USA* 2009; 106: 3645–3646.
47. Viboud C, Alonso WJ, Simonsen L. Influenza in tropical regions. *PLoS Med* 2006; 3: e89.
48. Reichelderfer P, Kendal A, Shortridge K, *et al.* Influenza surveillance in the Pacific Basin; seasonality of virus occurrence: a preliminary report. *In*: Chan YC, Doraisingham S, Ling AE, eds. Current Topics in Medical Virology. Singapore, World Scientific, 1989; pp. 412–444.
49. Yang L, Wong CM, Lau EHY, *et al.* Synchrony of clinical and laboratory surveillance for influenza in Hong Kong. *PLoS One* 2008; 3: e1399.
50. Maneewong P, Prasittikhet K, Pattamadilok S. Influenza virus isolation in Bangkok between 1988–1995. *J Health Sci* 2012; 6: 668–672.
51. Rao B, Banerjee K. Influenza surveillance in Pune, India, 1978–90. *Bull World Health Organ* 1993; 71: 177.
52. Doraisingham S, Goh KT, Ling AE, *et al.* Influenza surveillance in Singapore: 1972–86. *Bull World Health Organ* 1988; 66: 57–63.
53. Doraisingham S, Ling A. Patterns of viral respiratory tract infections in Singapore. *Ann Acad Med Singapore* 1986; 15: 9–14.
54. Alonso WJ, Viboud C, Simonsen L, *et al.* Seasonality of influenza in Brazil: a traveling wave from the Amazon to the Subtropics. *Am J Epidemiol* 2007; 165: 1434–1442.
55. Hall CE, Cooney MK, Fox JP. The Seattle virus watch: IV. Comparative epidemiologic observations of infections with influenza A and B viruses, 1965–1969, in families with young children. *Am J Epidemiol* 1973; 98: 365–380.
56. Davis LE, Caldwell GG, Lynch RE, *et al.* Hong Kong influenza: the epidemiologic features of a high school family study analyzed and compared with a similar study during the 1957 Asian influenza epidemic. *Am J Epidemiol* 1970; 92: 240–247.
57. Hayward AC, Fragaszy EB, Bermingham A, *et al.* Comparative community burden and severity of seasonal and pandemic influenza: results of the Flu Watch cohort study. *Lancet Respir Med* 2014; 2: 445–454.
58. Cox N. Enhancing influenza surveillance: from the global to local perspective. Presentation at the Institute of Medicine Workshop on Pandemic Influenza: Assessing Capabilities for Prevention and Response. Washington, Institute of Medicine Forum on Microbial Threats, 2004.
59. WHO. Global Epidemiological Surveillance Standards for Influenza. Geneva, World Health Organization, 2014.
60. WHO. Influenza (seasonal). Fact Sheet No. 211. Geneva, World Health Organization, 2009. www.who.int/mediacentre/factsheets/fs211/en/index.html
61. Su S, Fry AM, Kirley PD, *et al.* Survey of influenza and other respiratory viruses diagnostic testing in US hospitals, 2012–2013. *Influenza Other Respir Viruses* 2016; 10: 86–90.
62. Warren-Gash C, Smeeth L, Hayward AC. Influenza as a trigger for acute myocardial infarction or death from cardiovascular disease: a systematic review. *Lancet Infect Dis* 2009; 9: 601–610.
63. Farr W. Vital Statistics: a Memorial Volume of Selections From the Reports and Writings of William Farr. London, Royal Sanitary Institute, 1885.
64. Serfling RE. Methods for current statistical analysis of excess pneumonia-influenza deaths. *Public Health Rep* 1963; 78: 494.
65. Clifford RE, Smith J, Tillett HE, *et al.* Excess mortality associated with influenza in England and Wales. *Int J Epidemiol* 1977; 6: 115–128.
66. Choi K, Thacker SB. An evaluation of influenza mortality surveillance, 1962–1979. I. Time series forecasts of expected pneumonia and influenza deaths. *Am J Epidemiol* 1981; 113: 215–226.
67. Thompson WW, Comanor L, Shay DK. Epidemiology of seasonal influenza: use of surveillance data and statistical models to estimate the burden of disease. *J Infect Dis* 2006; 194: Suppl. 2, S82–S91.
68. Nicoll A, Ciancio B, Lopez Chavarrias V, *et al.* Influenza-related deaths – available methods for estimating numbers and detecting patterns for seasonal and pandemic influenza in Europe. *Euro Surveill* 2012; 17, 20162.
69. Fox JP, Hall CE, Cooney MK, *et al.* Influenzavirus infections in Seattle families, 1975–1979: I. Study design, methods and the occurrence of infections by time and age. *Am J Epidemiol* 1982; 116: 212–227.
70. Monto AS, Kioumehr F. The Tecumseh study of respiratory illness: IX. Occurrence of influenza in the community, 1966–1971. *Am J Epidemiol* 1975; 102: 553–563.
71. Chin TD, Mosley WH, Poland JD, *et al.* Epidemiologic studies of type B influenza in 1961–1962. *Am J Public Health Nations Health* 1963; 53: 1068–1074.
72. Philip RN, Bell JA, Davis DJ, *et al.* Epidemiologic studies on influenza in familial and general population groups, 1951–1956: characteristics of occurrence. *Am J Epidemiol* 1961; 73: 123–137.
73. Glezen WP, Couch RB, MacLean RA, *et al.* Interpandemic influenza in the Houston area, 1974–76. *N Engl J Med* 1978; 298: 587–592.
74. Tan Y, Guan W, Lam TT-Y, *et al.* Differing epidemiological dynamics of influenza B virus lineages in Guangzhou, southern China, 2009–2010. *J Virol* 2013; 87: 12447–12456.

75. Xu C, Chan K-H, Tsang TK, *et al.* Comparative epidemiology of influenza B Yamagata- and Victoria-lineage viruses in households. *Am J Epidemiol* 2015; 182: 705–713.
76. Ampofo K, Gesteland PH, Bender J, *et al.* Epidemiology, complications, and cost of hospitalization in children with laboratory-confirmed influenza infection. *Pediatrics* 2006; 118: 2409–2417.
77. Coffin SE, Zaoutis TE, Rosenquist ABW, *et al.* Incidence, complications, and risk factors for prolonged stay in children hospitalized with community-acquired influenza. *Pediatrics* 2007; 119: 740–748.
78. Poehling KA, Edwards KM, Weinberg GA, *et al.* The underrecognized burden of influenza in young children. *N Engl J Med* 2006; 355: 31–40.
79. Thompson WW, Shay DK, Weintraub E, *et al.* Influenza-associated hospitalizations in the United States. *JAMA* 2004; 292: 1333–1340.
80. Zhou H, Thompson WW, Viboud CG, *et al.* Hospitalizations associated with influenza and respiratory syncytial virus in the United States, 1993–2008. *Clin Infect Dis* 2012; 54: 1427–1436.
81. Public Health England. 2014. Surveillance of influenza and other respiratory viruses in the United Kingdom: Winter 2013/14. www.gov.uk/government/uploads/system/uploads/attachment_data/file/325203/Flu_annual_report_June_2014.pdf Date last accessed: December 21, 2015.
82. Mendez-Figueroa H, Raker C, Anderson BL. Neonatal characteristics and outcomes of pregnancies complicated by influenza infection during the 2009 pandemic. *Am J Obstet Gynecol* 2011; 204: S58–S63.
83. Pierce M, Kurinczuk JJ, Spark P, *et al.* Perinatal outcomes after maternal 2009/H1N1 infection: national cohort study. *BMJ* 2011; 342: d3214.
84. Morgan OW, Bramley A, Fowlkes A, *et al.* Morbid obesity as a risk factor for hospitalization and death due to 2009 pandemic influenza A(H1N1) disease. *PLoS One* 2010, 5: e9694.
85. Hayden F, Palese P. Influenza virus. *In*: Richmond DD, Whitley RJ, Hayden FG, eds. Clinical Virology. 3rd Edn. Washington, American Society for Microbiology Press, 2009; p. 943.
86. Widdowson M-A, Monto AS. Epidemiology of influenza. *In*: Webster RG, Monto AS, Braciale TJ, *et al.*, eds. Textbook of Influenza. 2nd Edn. Oxford, John Wiley & Sons, 2013; pp. 250–266.
87. Monto AS, Gravenstein S, Elliott M, *et al.* Clinical signs and symptoms predicting influenza infection. *Arch Intern Med* 2000; 160: 3243–3247.
88. Lee N, Ison MG. Diagnosis, management and outcomes of adults hospitalized with influenza. *Antivir Ther* 2012; 17: 143.
89. Jain S, Self WH, Wunderink RG, *et al.* Community-acquired pneumonia requiring hospitalization among U.S. adults. *N Engl J Med* 2015; 373: 415–427.
90. Gupta RK, George R, Nguyen-Van-Tam JS. Bacterial pneumonia and pandemic influenza planning. *Emerg Infect Dis* 2008; 14: 1187–1192.
91. Joseph C, Togawa Y, Shindo N. Bacterial and viral infections associated with influenza. *Influenza Other Respir Viruses* 2013; 7: 105–113.
92. Grabowska K, Högberg L, Penttinen P, *et al.* Occurrence of invasive pneumococcal disease and number of excess cases due to influenza. *BMC Infect Dis* 2006; 6: 1–9.
93. Bhat N, Wright JG, Broder KR, *et al.* Influenza-associated deaths among children in the United States, 2003–2004. *N Engl J Med* 2005; 353: 2559–2567.
94. McCullers JA. The co-pathogenesis of influenza viruses with bacteria in the lung. *Nat Rev Microbiol* 2014; 12: 252–262.
95. Simonsen L. The global impact of influenza on morbidity and mortality. *Vaccine* 1999; 17: S3–S10.
96. Nicholson K. Human influenza. *In*: Nicholson KG, Webster RG, Hay AJ, eds. Textbook of Influenza. Oxford, Blackwell Science, 1998, pp. 219–266.
97. Jacobs JH, Viboud C, Tchetgen ET, *et al.* The association of meningococcal disease with influenza in the United States, 1989–2009. *PLoS One* 2014; 9: e107486.
98. Mamas MA, Fraser D, Neyses L. Cardiovascular manifestations associated with influenza virus infection. *Int J Cardiol* 2008; 130: 304–309.
99. Smeeth L, Thomas SL, Hall AJ, *et al.* Risk of myocardial infarction and stroke after acute infection or vaccination. *N Engl J Med* 2004; 351: 2611–2618.
100. Muller MP, McGeer AJ, Hassan K, *et al.* Evaluation of pneumonia severity and acute physiology scores to predict ICU admission and mortality in patients hospitalized for influenza. *PLoS One* 2010; 5: e9563.
101. Myles PR, Nguyen-Van-Tam JS, Lim WS, *et al.* Comparison of CATs, CURB-65 and PMEWS as triage tools in pandemic influenza admissions to UK hospitals: case control analysis using retrospective data. *PLoS One* 2012; 7: e34428.
102. WHO Global Influenza Surveillance Network. Manual for the Laboratory Diagnosis and Virological Surveillance of Influenza. Geneva, World Health Organization, 2011.
103. Nicholson KG, Abrams KR, Batham S, *et al.* Randomised controlled trial and health economic evaluation of the impact of diagnostic testing for influenza, respiratory syncytial virus and *Streptococcus pneumoniae* infection on the management of acute admissions in the elderly and high-risk 18- to 64-year-olds. *Health Technol Assess* 2014; 18: 1–274.

104. Khandaker G, Heron L, Rashid H, *et al.* Comparing the use of, and considering the need for, lumbar puncture in children with influenza or other respiratory virus infections. *Influenza Other Respir Viruses* 2013; 7: 932–937.
105. Centers for Disease C, Prevention. Evaluation of 11 commercially available rapid influenza diagnostic tests – United States, 2011–2012. *MMWR Morb Mortal Wkly Rep* 2012; 61: 873–876.
106. Chartrand C, Leeflang MM, Minion J, *et al.* Accuracy of rapid influenza diagnostic tests: a meta-analysis. *Ann Intern Med* 2012; 156: 500–511.
107. Taubenberger JK, Morens DM. The pathology of influenza virus infections. *Annu Rev Pathol* 2008; 3: 499–522.
108. Krug RM, Aramini JM. Emerging antiviral targets for influenza A virus. *Trends Pharmacol Sci* 2009; 30: 269–277.
109. Hayden FG. Antivirals for influenza: historical perspectives and lessons learned. *Antiviral Res* 2006; 71: 372–378.
110. Ison MG. Clinical use of approved influenza antivirals: therapy and prophylaxis. *Influenza Other Respir Viruses* 2012; 7: 7–13.
111. Electronic Medicines Compendium. Relenza 5 mg/dose inhalation powder. 2015. www.medicines.org.uk/emc/medicine/2608
112. Electronic Medicines Compendium. Tamiflu 30 mg and 45 mg Hard Capsules. 2015. www.medicines.org.uk/emc/medicine/20294
113. Moscona A. Neuraminidase inhibitors for influenza. *N Engl J Med* 2005; 353: 1363–1373.
114. Kawai N, Ikematsu H, Iwaki N, *et al.* A comparison of the effectiveness of oseltamivir for the treatment of influenza A and influenza B: a Japanese multicenter study of the 2003–2004 and 2004–2005 influenza seasons. *Clin Infect Dis* 2006; 43: 439–444.
115. Jefferson T, Jones M, Doshi P, *et al.* Oseltamivir for influenza in adults and children: systematic review of clinical study reports and summary of regulatory comments. *BMJ* 2014; 348: g2545.
116. Dobson J, Whitley RJ, Pocock S, *et al.* Oseltamivir treatment for influenza in adults: a meta-analysis of randomised controlled trials. *Lancet* 2015; 385: 1729–1737.
117. Hsu J, Santesso N, Mustafa R, *et al.* Antivirals for treatment of influenza. *Ann Intern Med* 2012; 156: 512.
118. Muthuri SG, Venkatesan S, Myles PR, *et al.* Effectiveness of neuraminidase inhibitors in reducing mortality in patients admitted to hospital with influenza A H1N1pdm09 virus infection: a meta-analysis of individual participant data. *Lancet Respir Med* 2014; 2: 395–404.
119. Muthuri SG, Venkatesan S, Myles PR, *et al.* Impact of neuraminidase inhibitors on influenza A(H1N1)pdm09-related pneumonia: an individual participant data meta-analysis. *Influenza Other Respir Viruses* 2016; 10: 192–204.
120. Fry AM, Goswami D, Nahar K, *et al.* Efficacy of oseltamivir treatment started within 5 days of symptom onset to reduce influenza illness duration and virus shedding in an urban setting in Bangladesh: a randomised placebo-controlled trial. *Lancet Infect Dis* 2014; 14: 109–118.
121. Sugaya N. Widespread use of neuraminidase inhibitors in Japan. *J Infect Chemother* 2011; 17: 595–601.
122. Centers for Disease Control and Prevention. 2015. Use of antivirals: background and guidance on the use of influenza antiviral agents. www.cdc.gov/flu/professionals/antivirals/antiviral-use-influenza.htm Date last accessed: December 21, 2015.
123. Public Health England. 2015. PHE guidance on use of antiviral agents for the treatment and prophylaxis of seasonal influenza (2015–16). www.gov.uk/government/uploads/system/uploads/attachment_data/file/457735/PHE_guidance_antivirals_influenza_2015_to_2016.pdf Date last accessed: December 21, 2015.
124. Academy of Medical Sciences, Wellcome Trust. 2015. Use of neuraminidase inhibitors in influenza. Available from: www.acmedsci.ac.uk/policy/policy-projects/treating-influenza/ Date last accessed: December 21, 2015.
125. Takashita E, Meijer A, Lackenby A, *et al.* Global update on the susceptibility of human influenza viruses to neuraminidase inhibitors, 2013–2014. *Antiviral Res* 2015; 117: 27–38.
126. Li T, Chan M, Lee N. Clinical implications of antiviral resistance in influenza. *Viruses* 2015; 7: 4929–4944.
127. Lackenby A, Hungnes O, Dudman S, *et al.* Emergence of resistance to oseltamivir among influenza A (H1N1) viruses in Europe. *Euro Surveill* 2008; 13: 8026.
128. Whitley RJ, Boucher CA, Lina B, *et al.* Global assessment of resistance to neuraminidase inhibitors, 2008–2011: The Influenza Resistance Information Study (IRIS). *Clin Infect Dis* 2013; 56: 1197–1205.
129. Hauge SH, Dudman S, Borgen K, *et al.* Oseltamivir-resistant influenza viruses A (H1N1), Norway, 2007–08. *Emerg Infect Dis* 2009; 15: 155–162.
130. Kramarz P, Monnet D, Nicoll A, *et al.* Use of oseltamivir in 12 European countries between 2002 and 2007 – lack of association with the appearance of oseltamivir-resistant influenza A (H1N1) viruses. *Euro Surveill* 2009; 14: 19112.
131. Nicoll A, Ciancio B, Kramarz P. Observed oseltamivir resistance in seasonal influenza viruses in Europe interpretation and potential implications. *Euro Surveill* 2008; 13: 1854–1861.
132. McKimm-Breschkin JL. Influenza neuraminidase inhibitors: antiviral action and mechanisms of resistance. *Influenza Other Respir Viruses* 2013; 7: 25–36.
133. Boivin G. Detection and management of antiviral resistance for influenza viruses. *Influenza Other Respir Viruses* 2013; 7: 18–23.
134. Memoli MJ, Hrabal RJ, Hassantoufighi A, *et al.* Rapid selection of oseltamivir- and peramivir-resistant pandemic H1N1 virus during therapy in 2 immunocompromised hosts. *Clin Infect Dis* 2010; 50: 1252–1255.

135. Nguyen JT, Smee DF, Barnard DL, *et al.* Efficacy of combined therapy with amantadine, oseltamivir, and ribavirin in vivo against susceptible and amantadine-resistant influenza A viruses. *PLoS One* 2012; 7: e31006.
136. Perelson AS, Rong L, Hayden FG. Combination antiviral therapy for influenza: predictions from modeling of human infections. *J Infect Dis* 2012; 205: 1642–1645.
137. BioCryst pharma. 2014. Rapivab (peramivir injection). Prescribing information. Available from www.rapivab.com/prescribing-information Date last accessed: April 21, 2016.
138. Kohno S, Yen MY, Cheong HJ, *et al.* Phase III randomized, double-blind study comparing single-dose intravenous peramivir with oral oseltamivir in patients with seasonal influenza virus infection. *Antimicrobial Agents Chemother* 2011; 55: 5267–5276.
139. McLaughlin MM, Skoglund EW, Ison MG. Peramivir: an intravenous neuraminidase inhibitor. *Expert Opin Pharmacother* 2015; 1–12.
140. Hata A, Akashi-Ueda R, Takamatsu K, *et al.* Safety and efficacy of peramivir for influenza treatment. *Drug Des Devel Ther* 2014; 8: 2017–2038.
141. Ikematsu H, Kawai N. Laninamivir octanoate: a new long-acting neuraminidase inhibitor for the treatment of influenza. *Expert Rev Anti Infective Ther* 2011; 9: 851–857.
142. ClinicalTrials.gov registry. 2015. https://clinicaltrials.gov Date last accessed: November 30, 2015.
143. Marjuki H, Mishin VP, Chesnokov AP, *et al.* An investigational antiviral drug, DAS181, effectively inhibits replication of zoonotic influenza A virus subtype H7N9 and protects mice from lethality. *J Infect Dis* 2014; 210: 435–440.
144. Webster RG, Govorkova EA. Continuing challenges in influenza. *Ann NY Acad Sci* 2014; 1323: 115–139.
145. Baranovich T, Wong SS, Armstrong J, *et al.* T-705 (Favipiravir) induces lethal mutagenesis in influenza A H1N1 viruses in vitro. *J Virol* 2013; 87: 3741–3751.
146. Haque A, Hober D, Blondiaux J. Addressing therapeutic options for Ebola virus infection in current and future outbreaks. *Antimicrob Agents Chemother* 2015; 59: 5892–5902.
147. Furuta Y, Gowen BB, Takahashi K, *et al.* Favipiravir (T-705), a novel viral RNA polymerase inhibitor. *Antiviral Res* 2013; 100: 446–454.
148. Nagata T, Lefor AK, Hasegawa M, *et al.* Favipiravir: a new medication for the Ebola virus disease pandemic. *Disaster Med Public Health Prep* 2015; 9: 79–81.
149. Rossignol JF. Nitazoxanide: a first-in-class broad-spectrum antiviral agent. *Antiviral Res* 2014; 110: 94–103.
150. Haffizulla J, Hartman A, Hoppers M, *et al.* Effect of nitazoxanide in adults and adolescents with acute uncomplicated influenza: a double-blind, randomised, placebo-controlled, phase 2b/3 trial. *Lancet Infect Dis* 2014; 14: 609–618.
151. Ramos I, Fernandez-Sesma A. Modulating the innate immune response to influenza A virus: potential therapeutic use of anti-inflammatory drugs. *Front Immunol* 2015; 6: 361.
152. Lee N, Leo Y-S, Cao B, *et al.* Neuraminidase inhibitors, superinfection and corticosteroids affect survival of influenza patients. *Eur Respir J* 2015; 45: 1642–1652.
153. Rodrigo C, Leonardi-Bee J, Nguyen-Van-Tam JS, *et al.* Effect of corticosteroid therapy on influenza-related mortality: a systematic review and meta-analysis. *J Infect Dis* 2014; 212: 183–194.
154. Yang JW, Fan LC, Miao XY, *et al.* Corticosteroids for the treatment of human infection with influenza virus: a systematic review and meta-analysis. *Clin Microbiol Infect* 2015; 21: 956–963.
155. Fedson DS. Treating influenza with statins and other immunomodulatory agents. *Antiviral Res* 2013; 99: 417–435.
156. Mehrbod P, Omar AR, Hair-Bejo M, *et al.* Mechanisms of action and efficacy of statins against influenza. *BioMed Res Int* 2014; 2014: 872370.
157. Mair-Jenkins J, Saavedra-Campos M, Baillie JK, *et al.* The effectiveness of convalescent plasma and hyperimmune immunoglobulin for the treatment of severe acute respiratory infections of viral etiology: a systematic review and exploratory meta-analysis. *J Infect Dis* 2015; 211: 80–90.
158. INSIGHT FLU005 IVIG Pilot Study Group. INSIGHT FLU005: an anti-influenza virus hyperimmune intravenous immunoglobulin pilot study. *J Infect Dis* 2016; 213: 574–578.
159. Shriver Z, Trevejo JM, Sasisekharan R. Antibody-based strategies to prevent and treat influenza. *Front Immunol* 2015; 6: 315.
160. Miller RRI, Crossno P, Rice T, *et al.* ARDS Network registry 2009 pandemic influenza A (H1N1) infection patients with severe hypoxemia: outcomes in those treated with and without ECMO. *Am J Respir Crit Care Med* 2011; 183: A1638.
161. Noah MA, Peek GJ, Finney SJ, *et al.* Referral to an extracorporeal membrane oxygenation center and mortality among patients with severe 2009 influenza A(H1N1). *JAMA* 2011; 306: 1659–1668.
162. Australia and New Zealand Extracorporeal Membrane Oxygenation Influenza Investigators, Davies A, Jones D, *et al.* Extracorporeal membrane oxygenation for 2009 influenza A(H1N1) acute respiratory distress syndrome. *JAMA* 2009; 302: 1888–1895.
163. US Food and Drug Administration. 2011. Influenza: developing drugs for treatment and/or prophylaxis. www.fda.gov/downloads/drugs/guidancecomplianceregulatoryinformation/guidances/ucm091219.pdf Date last accessed: March 10, 2016.
164. Ison MG, de Jong MD, Gilligan KJ, *et al.* End points for testing influenza antiviral treatments for patients at high risk of severe and life-threatening disease. *J Infect Dis* 2010; 201: 1654–1662.

165. Nguyen-Van-Tam JS, Venkatesan S, Muthuri SG, *et al.* Neuraminidase inhibitors: who, when, where? *Clin Microbiol Infect* 2015; 21: 222–225.
166. Keitel WA, Neuzil KM, Treanor J. Immunogenicity, efficacy of inactivated/live virus seasonal and pandemic vaccines. *In*: Webster RG, Monto AS, Braciale TJ, *et al.*, eds. Textbook of Influenza. 2nd Edn. Oxford, John Wiley & Sons, 2013; pp. 311–326.
167. de Bruijn IA, Nauta J, Cramer WCM, *et al.* Clinical experience with inactivated, virosomal influenza vaccine. *Vaccine* 2005; 23: S39–S49.
168. Krammer F, Palese P. Advances in the development of influenza virus vaccines. *Nat Rev Drug Discov* 2015; 14: 167–182.
169. Pasquale A, Preiss S, Silva F, *et al.* Vaccine adjuvants: from 1920 to 2015 and beyond. *Vaccines* 2015; 3: 320–343.
170. Wiersma L, Rimmelzwaan G, de Vries R. Developing universal influenza vaccines: hitting the nail, not just on the head. *Vaccines* 2015; 3: 239–262.
171. Osterhaus A, Fouchier R, Rimmelzwaan G. Towards universal influenza vaccines? *Philos Trans R Soc Lond B Biol Sci* 2011; 366: 2766–2773.
172. Centers for Disease Control and Prevention. 2015. Vaccination: who should do it, who should not and who should take precautions. www.cdc.gov/flu/protect/whoshouldvax.htm Date last accessed: December 14, 2015.
173. Public Health England. Influenza. *In*: Immunisation Against Infectious Disease. London, Public Health England, 2015. www.gov.uk/government/uploads/system/uploads/attachment_data/file/456568/2904394_Green_Book_Chapter_19_v10_0.pdf Date last accessed: December 14, 2015.
174. Turner PJ, Southern J, Andrews NJ, *et al.* Safety of live attenuated influenza vaccine in young people with egg allergy: multicentre prospective cohort study. *BMJ* 2015; 351: h6291.
175. Marra F, Young F, Richardson K, *et al.* A meta-analysis of intradermal versus intramuscular influenza vaccines: immunogenicity and adverse events. *Influenza Other Respir Viruses* 2013; 7: 584–603.
176. Ansaldi F, de Florentiis D, Durando P, *et al.* Fluzone intradermal vaccine: a promising new chance to increase the acceptability of influenza vaccination in adults. *Expert Rev Vaccines* 2012; 11: 17–25.
177. Pebody R, Warburton F, Ellis J, *et al.* Low effectiveness of seasonal influenza vaccine in preventing laboratory-confirmed influenza in primary care in the United Kingdom: 2014/15 mid-season results. *Eurosurveillance* 2015; 20: 21025.
178. Ambrose CS, Levin MJ. The rationale for quadrivalent influenza vaccines. *Hum Vaccin Immunother* 2012; 8: 81–88.
179. Sridhar S, Brokstad K, Cox R. Influenza vaccination strategies: comparing inactivated and live attenuated influenza vaccines. *Vaccines* 2015; 3: 373–389.
180. DiazGranados CA, Dunning AJ, Kimmel M, *et al.* Efficacy of high-dose versus standard-dose influenza vaccine in older adults. *N Engl J Med* 2014; 371: 635–645.
181. Soema PC, Kompier R, Amorij J-P, *et al.* Current and next generation influenza vaccines: formulation and production strategies. *Eur J Pharm Biopharm* 2015; 94: 251–263.
182. Milián E, Kamen AA. Current and emerging cell culture manufacturing technologies for influenza vaccines. *BioMed Res Int* 2015; 2015: 504831.
183. Redkiewicz P, Sirko A, Kamel KA, *et al.* Plant expression systems for production of hemagglutinin as a vaccine against influenza virus. *Acta Biochim Pol* 2014; 61: 551–560.
184. Petrie JG, Ohmit SE, Johnson E, *et al.* Efficacy studies of influenza vaccines: effect of end points used and characteristics of vaccine failures. *J Infect Dis* 2011; 203: 1309–1315.
185. Kavanagh K, Robertson C, McMenamin J. Assessment of the variability in influenza A(H1N1) vaccine effectiveness estimates dependent on outcome and methodological approach. *PLoS One* 2011; 6: e28743.
186. Demicheli V, Jefferson T, Al-Ansary LA, *et al.* Vaccines for preventing influenza in healthy adults. *Cochrane Database Syst Rev* 2014; 3: CD001269.
187. Cates C, Rowe B. Vaccines for preventing flu in people with asthma. *Cochrane Database Syst Rev* 2013; 2: CD000364.
188. Valenciano M, Kissling E, Cohen J-M, *et al.* Estimates of pandemic influenza vaccine effectiveness in Europe, 2009–2010: results of influenza monitoring vaccine effectiveness in Europe (I-MOVE) multicentre case–control study. *PLoS Med* 2011; 8: e1000388.
189. Kissling E, Valenciano M, Falcao J, *et al.* "I-MOVE" towards monitoring seasonal and pandemic influenza vaccine effectiveness: lessons learnt from a pilot multi-centric case-control study in Europe, 2008–9. *Euro Surveill* 2009; 14: 19388.
190. Kissling E, Valenciano M, Cohen JM, *et al.* I-MOVE multi-centre case control study 2010-11: overall and stratified estimates of influenza vaccine effectiveness in Europe. *PLoS One* 2011; 6: e27622.
191. Kissling E, Valenciano M, I-MOVE Case–Control Studies Team. Early estimates of seasonal influenza vaccine effectiveness in Europe among target groups for vaccination: results from the I-MOVE multicentre case-control study, 2011/12. *Euro Surveill* 2012; 17: 20146.
192. Kissling E, Valenciano M, Larrauri A, *et al.* Low and decreasing vaccine effectiveness against influenza A (H3) in 2011/12 among vaccination target groups in Europe: results from the I-MOVE multicentre case–control study. *Euro Surveill* 2013; 18: 20390.

193. Kissling E, Valenciano M, Buchholz U, *et al.* Influenza vaccine effectiveness estimates in Europe in a season with three influenza type/subtypes circulating: the I-MOVE multicentre case-control study, influenza season 2012/13. *Euro Surveill* 2014; 19: 20701.
194. Valenciano M, Kissling E, Reuss A, *et al.* The European I-MOVE Multicentre 2013–2014 Case-Control Study. Homogeneous moderate influenza vaccine effectiveness against A (H1N1) pdm09 and heterogenous results by country against A (H3N2). *Vaccine* 2015; 33: 2813–2822.
195. Beyer WE, McElhaney J, Smith DJ, *et al.* Cochrane re-arranged: support for policies to vaccinate elderly people against influenza. *Vaccine* 2013; 31: 6030–6033.
196. Beck CR, McKenzie BC, Hashim AB, *et al.* Influenza vaccination for immunocompromised patients: systematic review and meta-analysis from a public health policy perspective. *PLoS One* 2011; 6: e29249.
197. Nokleby H, Nicoll A. Risk groups and other target groups – preliminary ECDC guidance for developing influenza vaccination recommendations for the season 2010-11. *Euro Surveill* 2010; 15: 19525.
198. European Centre for Disease Prevention and Control. 2016. Influenza vaccination. http://ecdc.europa.eu/en/healthtopics/seasonal_influenza/vaccines/Pages/influenza_vaccination.aspx Date last accessed: April 21, 2016.
199. Nicoll A, Ciancio B, Tsolova S, *et al.* The scientific basis for offering seasonal influenza immunisation to risk groups in Europe. *Euro Surveill* 2008; 13: 19018.
200. World Health Organization. Vaccines against influenza. WHO position paper – November 2012. *Wkly Epidemiol Rec* 2012; 87: 461–476.
201. Pebody R, Green H, Andrews N, *et al.* Uptake and impact of vaccinating school age children against influenza during a season with circulation of drifted influenza A and B strains, England, 2014/15. *Euro Surveill* 2015; 20; 30029.
202. Pebody R, Green H, Andrews N, *et al.* Uptake and impact of a new live attenuated influenza vaccine programme in England: early results of a pilot in primary school-age children, 2013/14 influenza season. *Euro Surveill* 2014; 19: 20823.
203. Carias C, Reed C, Kim IK, *et al.* Net costs due to seasonal influenza vaccination – United States, 2005–2009. *PLoS One* 2015; 10: e0132922.
204. Haber P. Guillain–Barré syndrome following influenza vaccination. *JAMA* 2004; 292: 2478.
205. Kwong JC, Vasa PP, Campitelli MA, *et al.* Risk of Guillain–Barré syndrome after seasonal influenza vaccination and influenza health-care encounters: a self-controlled study. *Lancet Infect Dis* 2013; 13: 769–776.
206. Vellozzi C, Iqbal S, Broder K. Guillain–Barre syndrome, influenza, and influenza vaccination: the epidemiologic evidence. *Clin Infect Dis* 2014; 58: 1149–1155.
207. Miller E, Andrews N, Stellitano L, *et al.* Risk of narcolepsy in children and young people receiving AS03 adjuvanted pandemic A/H1N1 2009 influenza vaccine: retrospective analysis. *BMJ* 2013; 346: f794.
208. Nohynek H, Jokinen J, Partinen M, *et al.* AS03 adjuvanted AH1N1 vaccine associated with an abrupt increase in the incidence of childhood narcolepsy in Finland. *PLoS One* 2012; 7: e33536.
209. European Medicines Agency. European Medicines Agency recommends restricting use of Pandemrix 2011. www.ema.europa.eu/docs/en_GB/document_library/Press_release/2011/07/WC500109182.pdf Date last accessed: December 12, 2015.
210. Pica N, Palese P. Toward a universal influenza virus vaccine: prospects and challenges. *Annu Rev Med* 2013; 64: 189–202.
211. Zhang H, Wang L, Compans R, *et al.* Universal influenza vaccines, a dream to be realized soon. *Viruses* 2014; 6: 1974–1991.

Acknowledgements: Thanks to Karl Albert Brokstad (University of Bergen, Bergen, Norway) for providing the figures.

Disclosures: J.S. Nguyen-Van-Tam reports employment by the following influenza vaccine or neuraminidase inhibitor manufacturers during the time periods stated: GlaxoSmithKline, 2000–2001; F. Hoffmann-La Roche, 2001–2002; and Aventis Pasteur MSD, 2002–2004. He has held no outstanding shares, share options or accrued pension rights in these companies since 2005. He has undertaken *ad hoc* consultancy and speaker honoraria from the following influenza vaccine or neuraminidase inhibitor manufacturers in the period 2008–2010: Sanofi-Pasteur MSD, Baxter AG, Solvay (Abbott), GlaxoSmithKline and F. Hoffmann-La Roche. He has current or recent research funding from F. Hoffmann-La Roche and GlaxoSmithKline, and has received travel expenses and congress registration fees from the European Scientific Working Group on Influenza (ESWI). P.R. Myles has received an unrestricted educational grant for pandemic influenza research from F. Hoffman-La Roche, travel expenses for a methodological seminar on evaluating antiviral effectiveness from Genentech, and travel expenses to deliver an evidence update on influenza antivirals to policy makers from ESWI.

Chapter 4

Avian influenza: H7N9, H5N1 and other novel strains

Hui Li[1] and Bin Cao[1,2]

Avian influenza (AI) viruses have caused great worldwide concern. So far, more than 13 strains of AI viruses have been shown to cross the species barrier and infect humans. Among them, the H5N1 and H7N9 strains have caused the highest mortality and morbidity worldwide. Clinical manifestations may range from asymptomatic, mild or moderate upper respiratory tract infection, to severe pneumonia and ARDS. Severe outcomes of AI infection in humans are the synergistic result of the intrinsic virulence of the virus and host factors. When treating severe AI infection, antiviral drug therapy is of great importance. However, drug resistance has emerged during treatment. More potent antiviral agents need to be isolated and investigated. In the meantime, ways to deal with the emergence of antiviral resistance, such as combining antiviral therapies with different modes of action, should be investigated. Immunopathology mediated by the inappropriate production of cytokines contributes to complicated influenza. Therefore, as well as antiviral drug therapy, the effectiveness of immunomodulators needs to be explored further.

Avian influenza (AI), more commonly known as "bird flu", refers to the infection caused by AI A viruses, which occur naturally among wild aquatic birds, but can infect domestic poultry and other animal species. AI viruses do not normally infect humans. However, sporadic human infection with AI viruses has been reported.

The history of AI viruses that cause infections in people can be traced back to 1959 [1]. Since then, more than 13 AI strains, including H7N9 [2], H5N1 [3], H7N7 [4], H4 [5], H5N2 [6], H5N6 [7], H7N2 [8], H7N3 [9], H9N2 [10], H6N1 [11], H10N7 [12], H10N8 [13], and H11Nx [14] have crossed the species barrier to infect humans. An apparent increase in reported cases of novel AI infections in humans has been observed in the past decade; this is partially due to the development of molecular diagnostic methods that have improved the detection of the AI virus. Another important factor that has contributed to the emergence of novel AI viruses is their high gene mutation and reassortment rate. Although most of the AI viruses isolated from humans so far cause mild or moderate illness, a few strains, particularly H5N1 and H7N9, have caused high mortality and morbidity. As of February 2015, more than 844 H5N1 confirmed cases from 16 countries and 571 H7N9 infected patients from China were reported to the World Health Organization (WHO), and the case

[1]Dept of Respiratory Medicine, Capital Medical University, Beijing, China. [2]Laboratory of Clinical Microbiology and Infectious diseases, Centre of Respiratory and Critical Care Medicine, China–Japan Friendship Hospital, Beijing, China.

Correspondence: Bin Cao, No. 2 Ying-hua Dong-jie, Chao-yang district, Beijing, 100029, China. E-mail: caobin_ben@163.com

 Print ISBN: 978-1-84984-069-9. Online ISBN: 978-1-84984-070-5. Print ISSN: 2312-508X. Online ISSN: 2312-5098.

fatality rates were 53.2% [15] and 37.1% [16], respectively. However, the case fatality rate reported to the WHO might not be a fair reflection of the much milder cases of H7N9 infection, as many mild cases of infection were not detected [17].

Although the cross-species and person-to-person transmission of AI viruses has been reported to be limited and insufficient [18], recent research found that some AI strains could be transmitted between mammalian species and even human beings by respiratory droplets [19–21]. In addition, specific mutations meant that AI viruses could spread easily between people, and novel influenza virus variants may emerge due to virus reassortment and the accumulation of mutations. Therefore, it is important to improve our pandemic preparedness.

This increase in novel zoonotic infections raises concern about the emergence of AI strains that could give rise to novel human pandemics. To step up vigilance, this chapter elucidates the virology, epidemiology, human pathogenesis, clinical characteristics, laboratory detection methods, diagnosis, and management of human infection by AI viruses, with an emphasis on the H5N1 and H7N9 strains. In addition, vaccination and prevention of AI virus infection are discussed briefly.

Virology

Avian influenza viruses

The influenza A virus is a single-stranded, negative-sense RNA virus, which belongs to the Orthomyxoviridae family of viruses. Its genome consists of eight separate gene segments surrounded by the lipid bilayer envelope. Influenza A viruses are divided into strains based on the antigenicity of two distinct glycoproteins that protrude from the lipid envelope, haemagglutinin (HA) and neuraminidase (NA). To date, 18 HA and 11 NA strains have been identified [22]. Among them, AI virus refers to the ones that naturally infect wild aquatic birds, but can sometimes cross the species barrier and infect domestic poultry and other animal species, including human beings [23].

Based on their ability to cause disease in poultry, AI viruses are divided into two groups: high-pathogenicity AI (HPAI) viruses or low-pathogenicity AI (LPAI) viruses. HPAI virus infection can cause severe disease, resulting in high mortality. By contrast, poultry infected with a LPAI virus may be asymptomatic or only present with mild illness, such as decreased egg production and depression [24, 25]. To date, most of the AI viruses isolated from humans belong to the LPAI category, including H6N1, H7N2, H7N9, H9N2, H10N7, H10N8, and some strains of H7N3 and H7N7, while two of the three AI virus strains infecting humans are HPAIs, namely H5N1 and H5N6.

Molecular determinants of virulence of avian influenza viruses

Up to 16 proteins are encoded by the AI virus genome [26, 27]. Among them, four influenza virus proteins, HA, polymerase basic protein 2 (PB2), nonstructural protein (NS1), and protein PB1-F2 are recognised as major determinants of virulence [25, 28]. Other proteins, such as polymerase acidic protein (PA) and polymerase basic protein 1 (PB1), also contribute to AI viral pathogenicity, while the function of other proteins has not yet been elucidated.

Haemagglutinin

The HA glycoprotein plays an important role in the initial stage of virus replication by mediating host-specific binding to sialic acid receptors on the cell surface. Its binding affinity for α2,6-linked and α2,3-linked sialic acid receptors is a major determinant of host tropism and transmission of influenza viruses. Human-derived viruses preferentially bind to α2,6-linked sialic acid; by contrast, AI viruses preferentially recognise α2,3-linked sialic acid receptors. However, α2,3-linked sialic acid receptors are expressed abundantly only on human nonciliated cuboidal bronchiolar cells of the lower respiratory tract, while α2,6-linked sialic acid is predominantly expressed on human epithelial cells of the upper respiratory tract [29]. Therefore, most natural strains of the AI virus cannot bind efficiently to human receptors to cause interspecies and/or human-to-human transmission at low doses. However, specific mutations in the HA receptor binding site could change the HA binding preference or allow enhanced and even efficient attachment to viral receptors of the α2,6-linked sialic acid kind on mammalian cells [30–34]. To date, most human AI virus isolates, including the recently identified strains of AI viruses, such as H6N1 [34], H7N9 [31], and H5N6 [35] have gained some adaptive mutations to human-type receptors, although they still retain an avian-type receptor preference. Only the H1, H2, and H3 strains have shifted receptor specificity from avian- to human-type and caused efficient transmissions in humans [36, 37].

Polymerase basic protein 2

PB2 is a major component of the influenza virus replication complex and is an important determinant of virulence. Evidence has shown that several genetic mutations of PB2 are related to host adaptation and the pathogenicity of AI viruses. Among them, the single mutation at the amino acid position 627 (E627K), which facilitates efficient replication of the AI virus in mammalian hosts, is the best characterised adaptation marker [38–40]. Naturally, AI virus isolates possess glutamic acid (E) at position 627, which restricts virus polymerase function in mammalian cells [41]. However, evidence has shown that another adaptive mutation of PB2 (D701N) can increase virulence and expand the host range of AI viruses to mammalian hosts by upregulating the binding ability of PB2, thus promoting the nuclear import of influenza viral ribonucleoprotein into mammalian cells [41]. A substantial number of H5N1 [38] and H7N9 virus isolates [42] and a small number of H7N7 strain [43] obtained from humans possess PB2-E627K or PB2-D701N substitutions. Recent research found that D701N and E627K mutations could emerge simultaneously and spontaneously in infected mammals and synergistically enhance the virulence of H7N9 [42].

Besides the well-characterised 627K and 701N loci, other adaptive mutations, such as the PB2-K526R substitution, have also been observed in a significant number of AI isolates from humans. PB2-K526R could also enhance viral replication in mammalian cells in combination with 627K [44].

Influenza nonstructural protein

NS1 is a homodimeric RNA-binding protein that has been implicated in a number of regulatory functions during AI virus infection. The most critical function revealed so far is its antagonism of IFN-α and β. This function may be achieved through several mechanisms. First, by blocking the recognition and signalling of molecular pattern receptors, such as cytoplasmic *retinoic inducible gene I* (*RIG-I*) [45–47] and TLR [48], NS1 could hinder IFN induction at the pre-transcriptional level. Second, NS1 has also been shown to inhibit the splicing, maturation [49], and exporting from the nucleus [50, 51] of host mRNAs, including IFN-β and IFN-responsive genes. Furthermore, research has revealed that NS1 with a NS1-D92E substitution is responsible for the resistance to antiviral cytokines of lethal AI H5N1 infection [52]. However, the mechanism of antiviral resistance of NS1 remains undetermined.

Protein PB1-F2

PB1-F2, which is encoded by the PB1 viral RNA segment in the +1 reading frame, was first discovered in 2001 in a study of CD8+ T-cell epitopes by CHEN *et al.* [53]. Since then, an increasing body of evidence has suggested that this multifunctional protein is related to an enhanced pathogenicity of the AI virus. PB1-F2 could enhance viral polymerase activity through its interaction with PB1 in a strain-specific manner [53–55]. However, some studies have indicated that PB1-F2 of some AI virus types could play a proapoptotic function in a cell type-dependent manner [53, 56]. Furthermore, PB1-F2 may also affect innate immune responses, inhibit the induction of IFN type I and promote inflammation by interacting with the adaptor protein mitochondrial antiviral-signalling protein [57, 58] and the NACHT, LRR and PYD domains-containing protein 3 inflammasome [59].

Epidemiology

Geographical distribution

At least 13 strains of the AI virus causing infections in humans have been reported so far. Among them, the H5N1 and H7N9 strains have caused large-scale outbreaks in humans and led to the highest morbidity and mortality rates. Sporadic human infections caused by the other AI virus strains, including H4Nx, H11Nx, H5N2, H5N6, H6N1, H7N2, H7N3, H7N7, H9N2, H10N7, and H10N8 have also been reported (table 1). However, no confirmed symptomatic H4Nx, H11Nx, and H5N2 human infection cases have been observed so far; these were proved by serological evidence alone. The geographical distribution of AI viruses is shown in table 1; the table outlines the geographical distribution of the AI viruses isolated from humans with an emphasis on the H5N1 and H7N9 strains.

The HPAI H5N1 virus was first isolated in 1996 from a farmed goose in the Guangdong province, China. The following year, it caused outbreaks in poultry in Hong Kong, China. However, it did not cause much concern until 1997, when 18 patients in Hong Kong were identified as infected with this virus, and six died because of it [3, 71]. No other confirmed H5N1 cases in humans were detected until 2003 in Southeast Asia. Since then, the HPAI H5N1 virus has evolved, with the emergence of multiple clades, and gained a long-term hold in these countries. Furthermore, it has continued its geographical migration from Southeast Asia to Eurasia and Africa [15]. As of February 2015, the H5N1 virus has migrated to at least 16 countries and more than 844 confirmed cases were reported to the WHO, with a case fatality rate of 53.2% [1, 5].

In April 2013, the first known human cases of infection with the H7N9 strain were reported in Shanghai and Anhui, China [2]. Unlike HPAI H5N1, this LPAI virus strain seems to more readily and quickly spread from animals to humans, although no evidence of efficient person-to-person transmission has been found. In the first 2 months after the initial report, the number of laboratory-confirmed H7N9 infections originating from these locations and several additional provinces, including Shandong, Zhejiang, Henan, Hunan, Fujian, Jiangxi, Jiangsu, Beijing, and Taiwan had already reached 132 [16, 72]. As of February 2015, three outbreaks of H7N9 among humans have been reported, and a total of

Table 1. Avian influenza (AI) virus strains that have caused human infections worldwide

AI virus	Source	Year and location of outbreak	Cases/ deaths n	Clinical features
H4				
H4Nx	Poultry	2007–2008, USA [5]; 2010, Lebanon [14]		Serological evidence only
H5				
A/H5N1	Poultry	1997, Hong Kong, China [3]; 2003–2015, 16 countries [15]	862/455	Pneumonia, diarrhoea
A/H5N2	Poultry	2005, Japan [6]		Serological evidence only
A/H5N6	Poultry	2014, Southern China [7]; 2015, Guangdong, China [60]	5/2#	ILI, pneumonia
H6				
H6N1	Unknown	2013, Taiwan, China [11]	1/0	Pneumonia
H7				
A/H7N2	Poultry, unknown	2002, Virginia, USA [61]; 2003, New York, USA [8]; 2007, UK [62]	6/0	ILI, pneumonia, conjunctivitis
A/H7N3	Poultry	2004, British Columbia, Canada [63]; 2006, Norfolk, UK [9]; 2012, Jalisco, Mexico [64]	5/0	Conjunctivitis
A/H7N7	Gull, poultry	1996, UK [4]; 2003, The Netherlands [65]; 2013, Italy [66]	93/1	Conjunctivitis, ILI, pneumonia
A/H7N9	Chicken, pigeon	2013–2015, China [16]	571/212	Pneumonia, ILI, diarrhoea
H9				
A/H9N2	Poultry	1999, Hong Kong, China [67]; 2003, Hong Kong, China [68]; 2011, Bangladesh [69]; 2013, Hunan, China [10]	10/0	ILI
H10				
A/H10N7	Duck, wild birds	2004, Ismailia, Egypt [12]; 2010, New South Wales, Australia [12]	9/0	ILI, conjunctivitis
A/H10N8	Poultry	2013, Jiangxi, China [13]	3/2	Pneumonia
H11				
H11Nx	Poultry, wild birds	2010, Lebanon [14]; 2004, USA [70]		Serological evidence only

#: case reported on 29 December 2015, in Guangdong, China. The patient remains in hospital.

571 laboratory-confirmed cases, including 212 deaths, have been reported to the WHO. Most of the cases originated from China, except for one Chinese traveller reported by Malaysia and two patients in Canada, who had travelled to China recently [16].

The remaining three AI virus strains identified in the past 2 years, including H5N6 [7], H6N1 [11], and H10N8 [13], have only caused sporadic infections in Southern China and no clusters were present. The three H10N8 cases were identified in the Jiangxi province of mainland China, while the five H5N6 cases were distributed in three different provinces of mainland China. First identified in February 2014, H5N6 infections in humans were detected in December 2015 in Guangdong, China [60]. Only one case of H6N1 infection in a human being has been reported so far.

Evidence for a zoonotic source

Epidemiological and molecular evidence suggests that poultry is the main source of most AI outbreaks in humans (table 1). Phylogenetic analysis has revealed that most AI viruses isolated from humans show a high similarity to the contemporary virus strains detected in live poultry [3, 11, 35, 61, 68, 73–75]. In some instances, large-scale outbreaks of AI occurred before or at approximately the same time as the emergence of human cases [3, 9, 62, 63, 66, 76]. Most of the human cases of AI virus infection reported so far have been poultry workers or individuals who had close contact with the affected animals [61, 65].

As for the H7N9 virus isolated from humans, evolutionary analyses have suggested that this is a reassortant virus strain of the H7 avian viruses and the enzootic H9N2 viruses [2]. The avian lineage from the H7N9 outbreak may have spread over a large geographic region, with live poultry markets as the main source of human infection [73, 77]. Data have suggested that more than 80% of H7N9 infected patients had a history of exposure to live animals, including waterfowl and chickens [78]. Epidemiological and molecular evidence has revealed that outbreaks of fatal AI H5N1 occurred in chicken farms in Hong Kong, just before the first human case was identified [79]. The sequence of human isolates showed high homology with the contemporary avian virus strains [80].

Person-to-person transmission

Most of the human cases reported so far have been scattered in different residential districts without apparent geographic clustering. However, a few family clusters have been reported for H7N9 [19, 78] and H5N1 [20, 21]. Therefore, person-to-person transmission of AI virus strains, particularly H5N1 and H7N9, can occur; however, transmission is inefficient and unsustainable. In addition, some researchers have suggested that adaptive mutations of the AI virus from wild birds to poultry may hinder human-to-human transmission. These adaptive mutations may include HAs with additional glycosylation sites impairing human receptor binding, increased pH of fusion resulting in environmental fragility, and NA stalk length truncation impairing the virus's ability to overcome the mucosal barrier [18]. Furthermore, the intrinsic host range restrictions of sialic acid receptor specificity and inadequate polymerase functions are barriers to the human-to-human transmission of AI viruses [29].

However, although such barriers make it difficult for the AI virus to readily spread among humans, one cannot exclude a situation where AI viruses might be able to adapt by means of reassortment and mutations.

Putative routes of transmission

AI viruses can be transmitted from poultry to human beings by inhalation of infectious droplets and aerosols *via* direct contact with sick poultry, or their infected blood or bodily fluids. Epidemiological data suggest that the highest transmission risk of H5N1 in humans is direct contact with poultry [81]. Some studies have demonstrated that AI viral RNA could be detected on various environmental surfaces or materials in influenza-associated households and their surroundings [82, 83]. However, it is still uncertain whether avian-to-human transmission might occur through an indirect route, such as exposure to contaminated water, cleaning poultry cages, or using poultry faeces as fertiliser. By contrast, several studies have reported that people might become infected with the AI virus through contact with the conjunctival mucosa [4], or *via* upper respiratory inoculation of contaminated water or fomites. Transmission of H5N1 through ingestion of infected poultry has been suspected in domestic cats [84].

Human pathogenesis

Strains of the AI virus, particularly H5N1 and H7N9, have been responsible for considerable morbidity and mortality worldwide, and are a serious concern to public health. The most common causes of death are viral pneumonia and ARDS [72]. Additionally, the most prominent histopathological features observed during autopsy were epithelial necrosis, diffuse alveolar damage, oedema, and intra-alveolar pulmonary haemorrhage [85, 86]. Although the main target organ in humans was the lung, biopsy from H5N1 infected individuals revealed that H5N1 could migrate beyond the lungs to the lymph nodes, gastrointestinal tract, liver, and brain [87]. By contrast, no viral infection was identified in extrapulmonary tissues or organs in the fatal H7N9 cases [86]. Pronounced histological changes, such as reduction of lymphoid tissue in the spleen, renal tubular degeneration, and spotty hepatic necrosis were observed in the *post-mortem* tissue samples collected from both H5N1 and H7N9 cases.

Extensive studies of animal models and influenza-infected patients have shown that high viral loads in the respiratory system and excessive proinflammatory responses were central to AI pathogenesis in human infections, particularly for the H5N1 and H7N9 strains. Accumulating data have shown that the levels of respiratory tract viral replication are associated with disease severity [88]. By contrast, reduction of viral load following antiviral treatment correlated with improved outcome [89, 90].

In addition to direct tissue destruction induced by viral replication, an exaggerated immune response has been associated with enhanced pathophysiology. In severe AI infections, innate and adaptive immune responses are activated in an attempt to control the virus. However, the immune responses might overreact to the virus resulting in the excessive production of proinflammatory cytokines and thereby aggravating the pathophysiology. In severe H5N1 and H7N9 infections, increased levels of cytokines and chemokines, such as macrophage migration inhibitory factor, stem cell factor, MCP-1, 10 kDa IFN-γ-induced protein, and IFN-γ were detected; these were positively related to disease severity and lung damage [88, 91–94]. Therefore, some experts have suggested using anti-inflammatory agents, such as sirolimus, chloroquine, and mesalazine, in combination with antivirals to inhibit the tissue damage resulting from the host immune response [95, 96]. Although controversial, some anti-inflammatory agents have been shown to be effective experimentally [97, 98].

Clinical manifestations

Symptoms and signs of avian influenza virus infection in humans

Humans infected with the AI virus were commonly asymptomatic or presented with mild, self-limiting illness. Occasionally, some strains of the AI virus might cause rapidly progressive pneumonia or ARDS and even death in humans. The frequency of severe outcomes was mainly determined by the virulence of the AI virus. LPAI virus infection, including H6N1, H7N2, H7N3, H9N2, and H10N7, usually caused mild-to-moderate symptoms and signs in humans, such as conjunctivitis, ILI, and sometimes pneumonia [9, 10, 12, 62]. The signs and symptoms of HPAI virus infection, including H5N1, H5N6, and H7N7, in people have been reported to range from conjunctivitis only, to ILI, to severe respiratory illness (*e.g.* shortness of breath, difficulty in breathing, pneumonia, ARDS, viral pneumonia, respiratory failure) with multiorgan disease [76, 99, 100]. However, this is not always the scenario. Although confirmed as having low pathogenicity in chickens, H7N9 has contributed to a considerable number of severe human infections and even deaths worldwide [72].

To date, subgroups of H5N1 and H7N9 have been responsible for the highest morbidity and mortality induced by AI virus infection worldwide. Usually, AI caused by H5N1 and H7N9 in humans starts with a fever, headache, and cough. A considerable number of patients subsequently deteriorate to progressive pneumonia and ARDS, while some cases are complicated by multiple organ failure and/or shock.

Laboratory findings of avian influenza virus infection in humans

Patients infected with the AI virus, particularly the H7N9 and H5N1 strains, usually have a normal or decreased leukocyte count. Wang *et al.* [101] observed that leukopenia, thrombocytopenia, and elevated alanine aminotransferase, creatinine kinase and lactate dehydrogenase were equally common in patients hospitalised with H7N9 and H5N1 infections. Wang *et al.* [101] also recorded lymphocytopenia in around 88 and 55% of patients hospitalised with H7N9 and H51N infections, respectively. Gao *et al.* [72] recorded elevated C-reactive protein (>10 $mg \cdot L^{-1}$) in >75% of patients hospitalised with H7N9 and H51N infections. In the study by Wang *et al.* [101], median C-reactive protein was 65 (25–113) $mg \cdot L^{-1}$ and 51 (14.2–118.3) $mg \cdot L^{-1}$ in patients hospitalised with H7N9 and H5N1 infections, respectively. In the study by Gao *et al.* [72], the majority of patients had a normal procalcitonin level, and $\leqslant$37% H7N9 hospitalised patients had a procalcitonin level >0.5 $ng \cdot mL^{-1}$.

Chest imaging features of patients with viral pneumonia induced by avian influenza

Consistent with histopathological changes [85, 86], in the pathogenic phase of the infection, the chest computed tomography (CT) scan of an individual with viral pneumonia induced by AI infection is characterised by ground-glass opacities, which may be accompanied by consolidation (figure 1a). With the deterioration of illness, partial and even areas of consolidation involving both lungs can be observed in some patients (figure 1b, c) [72, 102]. However, in the resolution phase, with the elimination of the proteinaceous exudate and inflammatory cells, the ground-glass opacities and consolidation shadows begin to resolve and are substituted by pulmonary fibroproliferative changes in some areas, which present as reticular shapes on the chest CT (figure 1d) [72].

Differences in clinical features between different strains of avian influenza

Although the clinical features of the different strains of the AI virus in humans share much in common, a few differences exist. Comparing the strains revealed that conjunctivitis was more common in the H7 strains including H7N2, H7N3, and H7N7 [62, 65], whereas in H5N1- and H7N9-infected patients, conjunctivitis had not been a feature. Diarrhoea has been inconsistently reported in H5N1 cases [71, 72, 100]. Compared with H5N1 cases, patients with H7N9 infection were much older, and a higher proportion was male. Diarrhoea

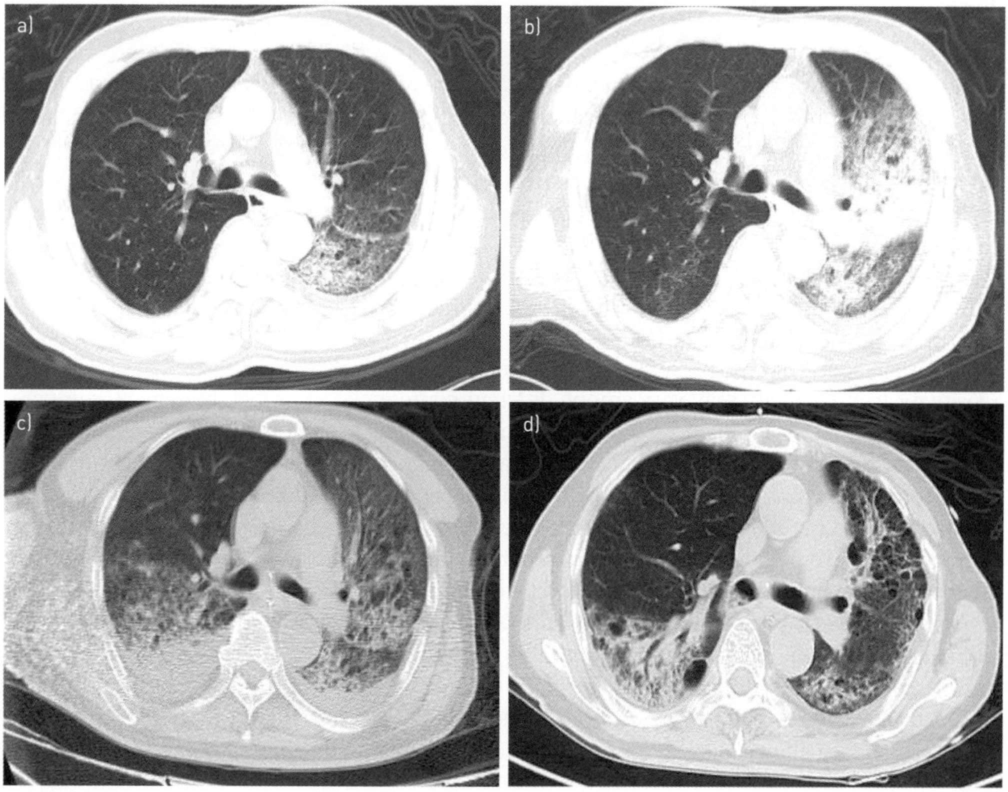

Figure 1. Chest computed tomography images from a 68-year-old man with pneumonia caused by the avian influenza A (H7N9) virus strain. a) Day 7 after the onset of illness: unilateral ground-glass opacities and partial consolidation can be seen in the upper and lower portions of the left lung, at the tracheal carina level. b) Day 9: rapid progression of the ground-glass opacities, along with consolidation in the left lung, can be observed. c) Day 16: increased ground-glass opacities in the left lung and increased consolidation in both lungs can be observed. d) Day 42: when the patient was discharged from hospital, ground-glass opacities and consolidation in both lungs had begun to resolve; predominant reticular changes and distortion of the previously involved areas of the parenchyma can be observed. Reproduced and modified from [72] with permission from the publisher.

or vomiting was reported in only 13.5% of H7N9 patients [72]. Underlying comorbidities were more common in H7N9 patients and duration of hospitalisation was longer for H7N9 patients [101].

Risk factors for a severe outcome

H7N9 caused high mortality in patients with a median age of 63 years. By contrast, symptoms seem to be mild in children. As part of China's national sentinel surveillance system for ILI, Ip *et al.* [17] identified that mild-to-moderate illness caused by the H7N9 virus strain could be detected in young patients with a mean age of 13 years (range: 2–26 years), and none had any underlying medical conditions. Multivariate logistic analysis revealed that age was a risk factor for severe outcomes for patients infected with the H5N1 or H7N9 strains [101, 103]. Underlying medical conditions, such as chronic heart disease, may be associated with high mortality in H7N9 patients [101]. The same results also apply to the H5N6 strain [7]. This indicates that, except for the intrinsic virulence of the AI virus, host factors are major contributors to a severe clinical outcome.

Laboratory detection of the avian influenza virus

Rapid identification of pathogens in infected patients is crucial to achieve the best clinical management, public health surveillance, and control outcomes. It is difficult to diagnose AI infections in humans based only on clinical characteristics. A study by Dugas *et al.* [104], based on a tertiary emergency department, revealed that clinical diagnosis has low sensitivity (<40%) for diagnosing influenza. Therefore, diagnostic tests are of great importance to help guide management in the clinical setting. To date, several diagnostic techniques are available, including RT-PCR, virus isolation in cell cultures or embryonated eggs, immunofluorescence detection of the virus in clinical specimens or isolates, rapid antigen tests, and other molecular techniques.

Sensitivity and specificity may vary among different commercial assay kits. In general, compared with conventional assays such as viral isolation, fluorescent detection, and rapid antigen tests, RT-PCR techniques are relatively rapid and have a higher sensitivity and specificity to detect and identify influenza viruses [105, 106]. Rapid antigen tests can detect an influenza virus in a qualitative way by identifying the viral nucleoprotein antigens in respiratory specimens. Although it has some advantages, such as providing quick results and being simple to perform, the technique is limited by the common occurrence of false negative results. Additionally, rapid antigen tests do not provide information on the specific strain of influenza A virus. Sometimes, antibodies detection from paired sera is also used to diagnose AI virus infection. Because convalescent serum is difficult to obtain, and because of time constraints (one sample taken during the first week of illness and another taken 3–4 weeks later), IgG antibody titre tests in paired sera are usually used as an epidemiological rather than a diagnostic tool.

Diagnosis of avian influenza virus infection in humans

The diagnosis of AI virus infection in humans should be based on clinical manifestations, history of contact, and virological tests. A probable case refers to a person with ILI, or an ARI and clinical, radiological, or histopathological evidence of pulmonary parenchymal disease (*e.g.* pneumonia or ARDS); the patient also has a history of close contact, in the 2 weeks before illness, with a laboratory-confirmed case of AI infection, or has travelled to any country or region where there was an ongoing influenza epidemic [107, 108]. Persons suspected of having an AI virus infection should undergo aetiological investigations, if available, for a definite diagnosis. Positive influenza A specimens whose strain cannot be established can be sent to a reference lab for confirmation [108]. A confirmed case is defined as a person with laboratory confirmation of a recent infection by PCR and/or viral isolation caused by a specific strain of the AI virus, such as H5N1, H7N9, and H5N6.

Management of avian influenza virus infections in humans

Antiviral drugs and potential immunomodulators

Antiviral drugs and drug resistance

Most of the data relating to antiviral drug therapy come from H7N9 and H5N1 infections; evidence for other strains of the AI virus isolated in humans is quite scarce. To date, two classes of antiviral drugs are commercially available: neuraminidase inhibitors (oseltamivir, zanamivir, peramivir, laninamivir); and M2-inhibitors (amantadine, rimantadine). Data on human AI infection, and *in vitro* experiments, revealed that the H7N9 virus strain is resistant to M2-inhibition because of the S31N mutation [109], while susceptibility to adamantanes for H5N1 viruses varied across regions, depending on the clade of virus in circulation [110, 111]. Therefore, M2-inhibitors are not recommended for use in severely ill A(H5N1) or A(H7N9) patients.

Neuraminidase inhibitors (NAIs), especially oseltamivir, are a standard therapy for viral pneumonia caused by infection with an influenza virus. Accumulative data suggest that NAIs, notably oseltamivir, can improve survival and reduce the incidence of a severe outcome [90, 112, 113], though its impact on viral shedding and reducing the duration of viral replication and transmission of the influenza virus remains controversial [114–116]. NAI antiviral therapy is not recommended as a routine therapy for otherwise healthy individuals with an uncomplicated clinical presentation induced by seasonal influenza or pandemic H1N1 [117, 118]. However, given the significant mortality associated with A(H5N1) and A(H7N9) infection, the WHO has recommended that oseltamivir should be prescribed as soon as possible when infection is suspected. Starting treatment should not be delayed by diagnostic testing [117].

Resistance to NAIs is an infrequent phenomenon, but some studies have suggested that secondary resistance might emerge during the course of therapy, resulting in viral load rebound and clinical progression [88, 90, 119]. Research has shown that the risk of antiviral resistance is especially high for immunocompromised patients, where prolonged viral shedding might be associated with the emergence of resistance-associated mutations [120].

Time, dose and duration of neuraminidase inhibitor therapy

Earlier initiation of NAI therapy results in a greater clinical benefit. Observational studies from seasonal and pandemic H1N1 influenza infection found an increase in the mortality hazard rate with each day's delay in initiating therapy. The benefit is greatest if NAI treatment is started within 2 days of the onset of illness [112, 121]. However, the therapeutic window is not limited to 2 days within the onset of illness. Although their magnitude was discounted, benefits were also found with later initiation of NAI therapy [112, 113, 116, 121–123]. In general, NAI treatment is indicated as early as possible for patients with confirmed or suspected AI virus infection. However, for some patients with prolonged viral replication, delayed antiviral treatment until 6–8 days of disease onset might prove beneficial.

As for the optimal dose and duration of NAI therapy in severe influenza infection, there is no consensus at the present time. One double-blind RCT and some observational studies have shown that no virological or clinical advantages were obtained from higher doses of oseltamivir therapy, when compared with the routine dose regimen [113, 124]. However, most of the data came from studies of seasonal or pandemic H1N1. In cases of severe H5N1 or H7N9 infection in humans, whether an increased dose provides greater antiviral effects needs to be investigated further. With regard to the duration of NAI treatment, to our knowledge, so far there have been no comparative studies. Some studies have suggested that the routine duration of oseltamivir treatment should be 5 days, while for clinically severe patients with complicated outcomes, the treatment could be prolonged based on the rate of viral clearance [125].

Immunomodulators and antiviral combinations for severe avian influenza virus infection

Recent studies have suggested that in some patients, particularly those infected with the H5N1 or H7N9 strains, even starting antiviral therapy early on could not inhibit disease progression. This might be explained by incompetent antiviral response, or drug resistance induced by single-drug antiviral therapy and immune-mediated injury, which could not be relieved by antiviral agents. Therefore, some researchers suggested combining antiviral drug therapy with different action modes and immunomodulators [126–128]. Although based on a sensible rationale, thus far few antiviral combinations have been tested in the clinical setting. As for combining antiviral drugs and immunomodulators, several studies have demonstrated that when combined with effective antiviral drugs, immunomodulators could prevent complications and decrease the mortality risk in some influenza patients [95, 97, 98, 121]. However, many immunomodulators are still at the experimental level and the controversy that surrounds them remains.

As potent modulators of the immune response, corticosteroids were widely prescribed for patients with severe influenza infection. However, accumulated evidence has shown that corticosteroids might not be beneficial and may even increase the risk of mortality [129, 130]. Findings from a recent meta-analysis of 16 observational studies revealed that corticosteroids had an overall harmful effect on populations affected by influenza [131]. An analysis of 288 patients infected with the H7N9 virus strain showed that high-dose corticosteroid therapy (>150 $mg \cdot day^{-1}$ methylprednisolone or equivalent) significantly increased both 30-day and 60-day mortality, while no significant impact was observed for low-to-moderate doses of corticosteroids (25–150 $mg \cdot day^{-1}$ methylprednisolone or equivalent) [132]. However, accurate conclusions could not be drawn from these observational studies because corticosteroids are generally given to patients with severe influenza. Furthermore, the dose, timing of initiation, and patients' disease severity and baseline immune conditions might all have an impact on the therapeutic effect of corticosteroids. In conclusion, so far the evidence from observational studies does not support combining antiviral drugs with corticosteroids. However, drawing a conclusion based on the evidence gathered so far is too arbitrary. Double-blind RCTs are needed.

Supportive care

Aside from antiviral treatment targeted at the influenza virus, appropriate supportive care is indispensable to improve the outcomes of patients with severe AI. The timely correction of hypoxaemia is of great importance, and oxygen saturation should be monitored as soon as possible and performed routinely during subsequent care. For patients with severe influenza and progressive hypoxaemia, as well as using standard noninvasive oxygen support methods, lung-protective mechanical ventilation (low tidal volume, low pressure), prone positioning ventilation, and extracorporeal membrane oxygenation should be performed appropriately [133]. For patients whose disease progression is complicated by shock, rescue therapy should be initiated timely and according to the appropriate guidelines [134].

Secondary infection and/or coinfection with pathogenic bacteria are important contributors to complicated outcomes in patients with pandemic or seasonal influenza infection [135]. Therefore, empirical antibiotic treatment has been suggested for influenza patients whose disease progression is complicated by pneumonia [136]. On admission, the most commonly isolated bacteria associated with severe pandemic H1N1 infection are *Streptococcus pneumoniae*, *Haemophilus influenzae* and *Staphylococcus aureus* [135]. As for H7N9 and H5N1, bacterial pathogens were isolated in about 16–25% of hospitalised patients; all the patients were hospitalised for at least 48 h with ventilator support [3, 71]. The most commonly observed bacteria were *Acinetobacter baumannii* and *Klebsiella pneumoniae* [71].

However, with regard to secondary bacterial pneumonia in AI infection cases, so far little evidence has been published. Given the high similarity between H5N1, H7N9, and pandemic H1N1 viral pneumonia, empirical antibacterial therapy has also been suggested; the choice of antibiotics should be based on the local guidelines for community-acquired pneumonia and on susceptibility patterns.

Vaccines and prevention of avian influenza infection in humans

As the principal measure to prevent infection and severe complications induced by the influenza viruses, vaccination is especially important for people at higher risk of serious complications (*e.g.* young children, pregnant women, and older people) and for people who live with or care for high-risk individuals. Evidence has shown that influenza vaccination could significantly reduce the risk of laboratory-confirmed influenza during sporadic, regional, and widespread outbreaks [137–139]. Influenza vaccination is also associated with reduced odds of hospitalisation for cases of laboratory-confirmed, influenza-associated pneumonia [140]. However, the protective efficacy of vaccination in the population has been assessed mainly for seasonal and pandemic H1N1 influenza vaccines. AI vaccines were tested for their immunogenicity. To date, a number of H5N1vaccines are available worldwide. These have been shown to elicit a strong, sustainable, and cross-clade immune response in the population [141, 142]. Nowadays, H5N1 vaccine supplies are kept as an emergency stockpile in some countries, in case of an outbreak of H5N1 infection among humans.

Except for vaccination, the best way to hinder human infection with AI viruses is to avoid any sources of exposure. Wild and domestic birds are the reservoir of a significant range of influenza viruses. Through reassortment and certain gene mutations, the AI viruses could spread from animals to human beings. The evidence so far has suggested that the predominant source of human infection is the live poultry market. A history of direct or close contact with poultry was reported in the majority of patients with AI virus infection [77]. Data from both the H5N1 and H7N9 strains has shown that closing live poultry markets could effectively decrease the risk of human infections with AI viruses [143, 144]. Some studies have also suggested that the implementation of frequent resting days in the live poultry/bird markets could also effectively reduce the transmission of AI viruses, though it is slightly less effective than the complete closure of markets [144, 145]. Other potential useful methods for reducing AI virus transmission include frequent cleaning and sterilising of poultry markets, strict control of third-party bird deliveries, and good hand hygiene [146].

Conclusion

AI viruses pose major threats to public health. In recent years, several novel AI viruses that can cross the species barrier to cause human infection have emerged. The live poultry markets are the main source of AI infection. Although some AI virus strains, because of a few adaptive mutations, have managed to spread from animal to human, AI viruses still have several barriers to overcome to be able to transmit from person to person efficiently. Because of the high mutation and reassortment rate of AI viruses, constant vigilance and surveillance are needed should more virulent and transmissible strains emerge. Most patients with an AI infection are asymptomatic or present with mild-to-moderate symptoms and signs, such as conjunctivitis and ILI (including cough, fever, sore throat, and headache). However, a significant number of patients infected with the H5N1 or H7N9 strains may progress to severe pneumonia, which may be complicated by ARDS, multiple organ failure, and/or shock. Viral replication and immune-mediated damage are responsible for the pathogenesis of AI infection in humans, especially in severe cases. To date, most AI viruses are sensitive to NAI treatment; however, a few resistant virus strains produced as the result of single-drug antiviral therapy have been detected. Combining antiviral therapy with different modes of action has been suggested; however, this needs to be explored with further experimental and clinical data. Immunomodulators in combination with antiviral drugs have been used to relieve the immunopathology of AI. However, they are still at the experimental stage. As for preventing AI infection in humans, except for vaccinating those who are at high risk of AI infection, direct or close contact with live poultry should be avoided.

References

1. Alexander DJ. Avian influenza viruses and human health. *Dev Biol (Basel)* 2006; 124: 77–84.
2. Gao R, Cao B, Hu Y, *et al.* Human infection with a novel avian-origin influenza A (H7N9) virus. *N Engl J Med* 2013; 368: 1888–1897.
3. Chan PK. Outbreak of avian influenza A (H5N1) virus infection in Hong Kong in 1997. *Clin Infect Dis* 2002; 34: Suppl. 2, 58–64.
4. Kurtz J, Manvell RJ, Banks J. Avian influenza virus isolated from a woman with conjunctivitis. *Lancet* 1996; 348: 901–902.
5. Kayali G, Ortiz EJ, Chorazy ML, *et al.* Evidence of previous avian influenza infection among US turkey workers. *Zoonoses Public Health* 2010; 57: 265–272.
6. Ogata T, Yamazaki Y, Okabe N, *et al.* Human H5N2 avian influenza infection in Japan and the factors associated with high H5N2-neutralizing antibody titer. *J Epidemiol* 2008; 18: 160–166.
7. Chen T, Zhang R. Symptoms seem to be mild in children infected with avian influenza A (H5N6) and other subtypes. *J Infect* 2015; 71: 702–703.
8. Ostrowsky B, Huang A, Terry W, *et al.* Low pathogenic avian influenza A (H7N2) virus infection in immunocompromised adult, New York, USA, 2003. *Emerg Infect Dis* 2012; 18: 1128–1131.
9. Nguyen-Van-Tam JS, Nair P, Acheson P, *et al.* Outbreak of low pathogenicity H7N3 avian influenza in UK, including associated case of human conjunctivitis. *Euro Surveill* 2006; 11: E060504.2.
10. Huang Y, Li X, Zhang H, *et al.* Human infection with an avian influenza A (H9N2) virus in the middle region of China. *J Med Virol* 2015; 87: 1641–1648.
11. Shi W, Shi Y, Wu Y, *et al.* Origin and molecular characterization of the human-infecting H6N1 influenza virus in Taiwan. *Protein Cell* 2013; 4: 846–853.
12. Arzey GG, Kirkland PD, Arzey KE, *et al.* Influenza virus A (H10N7) in chickens and poultry abattoir workers, Australia. *Emerg Infect Dis* 2012; 18: 814–816.
13. Chen S, Li Z, Hu M, *et al.* Knowledge, attitudes, and practices (KAP) relating to avian influenza (H10N8) among farmers' markets workers in Nanchang, China. *PLoS One* 2015; 10: e0127120.
14. Kayali G, Barbour E, Dbaibo G, *et al.* Evidence of infection with H4 and H11 avian influenza viruses among Lebanese chicken growers. *PLoS One* 2011; 6: e26818.
15. World Health Organization. Influenza at the Human-Animal Interface (HAI). Cumulative number of confirmed human cases for avian influenza A(H5N1) reported to WHO, 2003–2015. www.who.int/influenza/human_animal_interface/EN_GIP_20151113cumulativeNumberH5N1cases.pdf?ua=1 Date last accessed: March 14, 2016. Date last updated: November 13, 2015.
16. World Health Organization. WHO risk assessment of human infections with avian influenza A(H7N9) virus. www.who.int/influenza/human_animal_interface/influenza_h7n9/RiskAssessment_H7N9_23Feb20115.pdf Date last accessed: March 14, 2016. Date last updated: February 23, 2015.
17. Ip DK, Liao Q, Wu P, *et al.* Detection of mild to moderate influenza A/H7N9 infection by China's national sentinel surveillance system for influenza-like illness: case series. *BMJ* 2013; 346: f3693.
18. Long JS, Benfield CT, Barclay WS. One-way trip: influenza virus' adaptation to gallinaceous poultry may limit its pandemic potential. *Bioessays* 2015; 37: 204–212.
19. Qi X, Qian YH, Bao CJ, *et al.* Probable person to person transmission of novel avian influenza A (H7N9) virus in Eastern China, 2013: epidemiological investigation. *BMJ* 2013; 347: f4752.
20. Wang H, Feng Z, Shu Y, *et al.* Probable limited person-to-person transmission of highly pathogenic avian influenza A (H5N1) virus in China. *Lancet* 2008; 371: 1427–1434.
21. Ungchusak K, Auewarakul P, Dowell SF, *et al.* Probable person-to-person transmission of avian influenza A (H5N1). *N Engl J Med* 2005; 352: 333–340.

22. Centers for Disease Control and Prevention. Influenza type A viruses. www.cdc.gov/flu/avianflu/influenza-a-virus-subtypes.htm Date last accessed: March 14, 2016. Date last updated: February 9, 2015.
23. Centers for Disease Control and Prevention. Information on avian influenza. www.cdc.gov/flu/avianflu/index.htm Date last accessed: March 14, 2016. Date last updated: July 23, 2015.
24. Swayne DE, Suarez DL. Highly pathogenic avian influenza. *Rev Sci Tech* 2000; 19: 463–482.
25. Neumann G, Chen H, Gao GF, *et al.* H5N1 influenza viruses: outbreaks and biological properties. *Cell Res* 2010; 20: 51–61.
26. Jagger BW, Wise HM, Kash JC, *et al.* An overlapping protein-coding region in influenza A virus segment 3 modulates the host response. *Science* 2012; 337: 199–204.
27. Muramoto Y, Noda T, Kawakami E, *et al.* Identification of novel influenza A virus proteins translated from PA mRNA. *J Virol* 2013; 87: 2455–2462.
28. Schrauwen EJ, de Graaf M, Herfst S, *et al.* Determinants of virulence of influenza A virus. *Eur J Clin Microbiol Infect Dis* 2014; 33: 479–490.
29. Shinya K, Ebina M, Yamada S, *et al.* Avian flu: influenza virus receptors in the human airway. *Nature* 2006; 440: 435–436.
30. Xiong X, Coombs PJ, Martin SR, *et al.* Receptor binding by a ferret-transmissible H5 avian influenza virus. *Nature* 2013; 497: 392–396.
31. Xiong X, Martin SR, Haire LF, *et al.* Receptor binding by an H7N9 influenza virus from humans. *Nature* 2013; 499: 496–499.
32. Sang X, Wang A, Ding J, *et al.* Adaptation of H9N2 AIV in guinea pigs enables efficient transmission by direct contact and inefficient transmission by respiratory droplets. *Sci Rep* 2015; 5: 15928.
33. Wang F, Qi J, Bi Y, *et al.* Adaptation of avian influenza A (H6N1) virus from avian to human receptor-binding preference. *EMBO J* 2015; 34: 1661–1673.
34. Tzarum N, de Vries RP, Zhu X, *et al.* Structure and receptor binding of the hemagglutinin from a human H6N1 influenza virus. *Cell Host Microbe* 2015; 17: 369–376.
35. Pan M, Gao R, Lv Q, *et al.* Human infection with a novel, highly pathogenic avian influenza A (H5N6) virus: virological and clinical findings. *J Infect* 2016; 72: 52–59.
36. Connor RJ, Kawaoka Y, Webster RG, *et al.* Receptor specificity in human, avian, and equine H2 and H3 influenza virus isolates. *Virology* 1994; 205: 17–23.
37. de Graaf M, Fouchier RA. Role of receptor binding specificity in influenza A virus transmission and pathogenesis. *EMBO J* 2014; 33: 823–841.
38. Hatta M, Gao P, Halfmann P, *et al.* Molecular basis for high virulence of Hong Kong H5N1 influenza A viruses. *Science* 2001; 293: 1840–1842.
39. Labadie K, Dos Santos Afonso E, Rameix-Welti MA, *et al.* Host-range determinants on the PB2 protein of influenza A viruses control the interaction between the viral polymerase and nucleoprotein in human cells. *Virology* 2007; 362: 271–282.
40. Massin P, van der Werf S, Naffakh N. Residue 627 of PB2 is a determinant of cold sensitivity in RNA replication of avian influenza viruses. *J Virol* 2001; 75: 5398–5404.
41. Subbarao EK, London W, Murphy BR. A single amino acid in the PB2 gene of influenza A virus is a determinant of host range. *J Virol* 1993; 67: 1761–1764.
42. Zhu W, Li L, Yan Z, *et al.* Dual E627K and D701N mutations in the PB2 protein of A(H7N9) influenza virus increased its virulence in mammalian models. *Sci Rep* 2015; 5: 14170.
43. de Wit E, Munster VJ, van Riel D, *et al.* Molecular determinants of adaptation of highly pathogenic avian influenza H7N7 viruses to efficient replication in the human host. *J Virol* 2010; 84: 1597–1606.
44. Song W, Wang P, Mok BW, *et al.* The K526R substitution in viral protein PB2 enhances the effects of E627K on influenza virus replication. *Nat Commun* 2014; 5: 5509.
45. Pichlmair A, Schulz O, Tan CP, *et al.* RIG-I-mediated antiviral responses to single-stranded RNA bearing 5′-phosphates. *Science* 2006; 314: 997–1001.
46. Mibayashi M, Martínez-Sobrido L, Loo YM, *et al.* Inhibition of retinoic acid-inducible gene I-mediated induction of beta interferon by the NS1 protein of influenza A virus. *J Virol* 2007; 81: 514–524.
47. Gack MU, Albrecht RA, Urano T, *et al.* Influenza A virus NS1 targets the ubiquitin ligase TRIM25 to evade recognition by the host viral RNA sensor RIG-I. *Cell Host Microbe* 2009; 5: 439–449.
48. Akira S. TLR signaling. *Curr Top Microbiol Immunol* 2006; 311: 1–16.
49. Nemeroff ME, Barabino SM, Li Y, *et al.* Influenza virus NS1 protein interacts with the cellular 30 kDa subunit of CPSF and inhibits 3′ end formation of cellular pre-mRNAs. *Mol Cell* 1998; 1: 991–1000.
50. Chen Z, Li Y, Krug RM. Influenza A virus NS1 protein targets poly(A)-binding protein II of the cellular 3′-end processing machinery. *EMBO J* 1999; 18: 2273–2283.
51. Satterly N, Tsai PL, van Deursen J, *et al.* Influenza virus targets the mRNA export machinery and the nuclear pore complex. *Proc Natl Acad Sci USA* 2007; 104: 1853–1858.
52. Seo SH, Hoffmann E, Webster RG. Lethal H5N1 influenza viruses escape host anti-viral cytokine responses. *Nat Med* 2002; 8: 950–954.

53. Chen W, Calvo PA, Malide D, *et al.* A novel influenza A virus mitochondrial protein that induces cell death. *Nat Med* 2001; 7: 1306–1312.
54. McAuley JL, Chipuk JE, Boyd KL, *et al.* PB1-F2 proteins from H5N1 and 20 century pandemic influenza viruses cause immunopathology. *PLoS Pathog* 2010; 6: e1001014.
55. Mazur I, Anhlan D, Mitzner D, *et al.* The proapoptotic influenza A virus protein PB1-F2 regulates viral polymerase activity by interaction with the PB1 protein. *Cell Microbiol* 2008; 10: 1140–1152.
56. Zamarin D, García-Sastre A, Xiao X, *et al.* Influenza virus PB1-F2 protein induces cell death through mitochondrial ANT3 and VDAC1. *PLoS Pathog* 2005; 1: e4.
57. Varga ZT, Ramos I, Hai R, *et al.* The influenza virus protein PB1-F2 inhibits the induction of type I interferon at the level of the MAVS adaptor protein. *PLoS Pathog* 2011; 7: e1002067.
58. Varga ZT, Grant A, Manicassamy B, *et al.* Influenza virus protein PB1-F2 inhibits the induction of type I interferon by binding to MAVS and decreasing mitochondrial membrane potential. *J Virol* 2012; 86: 8359–8366.
59. McAuley JL, Tate MD, MacKenzie-Kludas CJ, *et al.* Activation of the NLRP3 inflammasome by IAV virulence protein PB1-F2 contributes to severe pathophysiology and disease. *PLoS Pathog* 2013; 9: e1003392.
60. Report of Health and Family Planning Commission of Guangdong Province, 2015. http://en.nhfpc.gov.cn/2015-06/03/c_46242.htm
61. Abdelwhab EM, Veits J, Mettenleiter TC. Prevalence and control of H7 avian influenza viruses in birds and humans. *Epidemiol Infect* 2014; 142: 896–920.
62. Avian influenza A/(H7N2) outbreak in the United Kingdom. *Euro Surveill* 2007; 12: E070531.2.
63. Tweed SA, Skowronski DM, David ST, *et al.* Human illness from avian influenza H7N3, British Columbia. *Emerg Infect Dis* 2004; 10: 2196–2199.
64. Centers for Disease Control and Prevention (CDC). Notes from the field: Highly pathogenic avian influenza A (H7N3) virus infection in two poultry workers – Jalisco, Mexico, July 2012. *MMWR Morb Mortal Wkly Rep* 2012; 61: 726–727.
65. Koopmans M, Wilbrink B, Conyn M, *et al.* Transmission of H7N7 avian influenza A virus to human beings during a large outbreak in commercial poultry farms in the Netherlands. *Lancet* 2004; 363: 587–593.
66. Puzelli S, Rossini G, Facchini M, *et al.* Human infection with highly pathogenic A(H7N7) avian influenza virus, Italy, 2013. *Emerg Infect Dis* 2014; 20: 1745–1749.
67. Peiris M, Yuen KY, Leung CW, *et al.* Human infection with influenza H9N2. *Lancet* 1999; 354: 916–917.
68. Butt KM, Smith GJ, Chen H, *et al.* Human infection with an avian H9N2 influenza A virus in Hong Kong in 2003. *J Clin Microbiol* 2005; 43: 5760–5767.
69. Shanmuganatham K, Feeroz MM, Jones-Engel L, *et al.* Antigenic and molecular characterization of avian influenza A(H9N2) viruses, Bangladesh. *Emerg Infect Dis* 2013; 19. DOI: 10.3201/eid1909.130336.
70. Gill JS, Webby R, Gilchrist MJ, *et al.* Avian influenza among waterfowl hunters and wildlife professionals. *Emerg Infect Dis* 2006; 12: 1284–1286.
71. Yuen KY, Chan PK, Peiris M, *et al.* Clinical features and rapid viral diagnosis of human disease associated with avian influenza A H5N1 virus. *Lancet* 1998; 351: 467–471.
72. Gao HN, Lu HZ, Cao B, *et al.* Clinical findings in 111 cases of influenza A (H7N9) virus infection. *N Engl J Med* 2013; 368: 2277–2285.
73. Lam TT, Wang J, Shen Y, *et al.* The genesis and source of the H7N9 influenza viruses causing human infections in China. *Nature* 2013; 502: 241–244.
74. Mok CK, Da Guan W, Liu XQ, *et al.* Genetic characterization of highly pathogenic avian influenza A(H5N6) virus, Guangdong, China. *Emerg Infect Dis* 2015; 21: 2268–2271.
75. Yuan J, Zhang L, Kan X, *et al.* Origin and molecular characteristics of a novel 2013 avian influenza A(H6N1) virus causing human infection in Taiwan. *Clin Infect Dis* 2013; 57: 1367–1368.
76. Fouchier RA, Schneeberger PM, Rozendaal FW, *et al.* Avian influenza A virus (H7N7) associated with human conjunctivitis and a fatal case of acute respiratory distress syndrome. *Proc Natl Acad Sci USA* 2004; 101: 1356–1361.
77. Ling F, Chen E, Liu Q, *et al.* Hypothesis on the source, transmission and characteristics of infection of avian influenza A (H7N9) virus–based on analysis of field epidemiological investigation and gene sequence analysis. *Zoonoses Public Health* 2015; 62: 29–37.
78. Li Q, Zhou L, Zhou M, *et al.* Epidemiology of human infections with avian influenza A(H7N9) virus in China. *N Engl J Med* 2014; 370: 520–532.
79. Shortridge KF. Poultry and the influenza H5N1 outbreak in Hong Kong, 1997: abridged chronology and virus isolation. *Vaccine* 1999; 17: Suppl. 1, 26–29.
80. Claas EC, Osterhaus AD, van Beek R, *et al.* Human influenza A H5N1 virus related to a highly pathogenic avian influenza virus. *Lancet* 1998; 351: 472–477.
81. Van Kerkhove MD. Brief literature review for the WHO global influenza research agenda–highly pathogenic avian influenza H5N1 risk in humans. *Influenza Other Respir Viruses* 2013; 7: Suppl. 2, 26–33.
82. Vong S, Ly S, Mardy S, *et al.* Environmental contamination during influenza A virus (H5N1) outbreaks, Cambodia, 2006. *Emerg Infect Dis* 2008; 14: 1303–1305.

83. Gutiérrez RA, Buchy P. Contaminated soil and transmission of influenza virus (H5N1). *Emerg Infect Dis* 2012; 18: 1530–1532.
84. Kuiken T, Rimmelzwaan G, van Riel D, *et al.* Avian H5N1 influenza in cats. *Science* 2004; 306: 241.
85. Korteweg C, Gu J. Pathology, molecular biology, and pathogenesis of avian influenza A (H5N1) infection in humans. *Am J Pathol* 2008; 172: 1155–1170.
86. Yu L, Wang Z, Chen Y, *et al.* Clinical, virological, and histopathological manifestations of fatal human infections by avian influenza A(H7N9) virus. *Clin Infect Dis* 2013; 57: 1449–1457.
87. Gu J, Xie Z, Gao Z, *et al.* H5N1 infection of the respiratory tract and beyond: a molecular pathology study. *Lancet* 2007; 370: 1137–1145.
88. de Jong MD, Simmons CP, Thanh TT, *et al.* Fatal outcome of human influenza A (H5N1) is associated with high viral load and hypercytokinemia. *Nat Med* 2006; 12: 1203–1207.
89. Kitano M, Itoh Y, Ishigaki H, *et al.* Efficacy of repeated intravenous administration of peramivir against highly pathogenic avian influenza A (H5N1) virus in cynomolgus macaques. *Antimicrob Agents Chemother* 2014; 58: 4795–4803.
90. Hu Y, Lu S, Song Z, *et al.* Association between adverse clinical outcome in human disease caused by novel influenza A H7N9 virus and sustained viral shedding and emergence of antiviral resistance. *Lancet* 2013; 381: 2273–2279.
91. Guo J, Huang F, Liu J, *et al.* The serum profile of hypercytokinemia factors identified in H7N9-infected patients can predict fatal outcomes. *Sci Rep* 2015; 5: 10942.
92. Huang R, Zhang L, Gu Q, *et al.* Profiles of acute cytokine and antibody responses in patients infected with avian influenza A H7N9. *PLoS One* 2014; 9: e101788.
93. Zeng H, Belser JA, Goldsmith CS, *et al.* A(H7N9) virus results in early induction of proinflammatory cytokine responses in both human lung epithelial and endothelial cells and shows increased human adaptation compared with avian H5N1 virus. *J Virol* 2015; 89: 4655–4667.
94. Shen Z, Chen Z, Li X, *et al.* Host immunological response and factors associated with clinical outcome in patients with the novel influenza A H7N9 infection. *Clin Microbiol Infect* 2014; 20: O493–O500.
95. Zumla A, Memish ZA, Maeurer M, *et al.* Emerging novel and antimicrobial-resistant respiratory tract infections: new drug development and therapeutic options. *Lancet Infect Dis* 2014; 14: 1136–1149.
96. Ramos I, Fernandez-Sesma A. Modulating the innate immune response to influenza A virus: potential therapeutic use of anti-inflammatory drugs. *Front Immunol* 2015; 6: 361.
97. Wang CH, Chung FT, Lin SM, *et al.* Adjuvant treatment with a mammalian target of rapamycin inhibitor, sirolimus, and steroids improves outcomes in patients with severe H1N1 pneumonia and acute respiratory failure. *Crit Care Med* 2014; 42: 313–321.
98. Yan Y, Zou Z, Sun Y, *et al.* Anti-malaria drug chloroquine is highly effective in treating avian influenza A H5N1 virus infection in an animal model. *Cell Res* 2013; 23: 300–302.
99. Yang ZF, Mok CK, Peiris JS, *et al.* Human infection with a novel avian influenza A(H5N6) virus. *N Engl J Med* 2015; 373: 487–489.
100. Tran TH, Nguyen TL, Nguyen TD, *et al.* Avian influenza A (H5N1) in 10 patients in Vietnam. *N Engl J Med* 2004; 350: 1179–1188.
101. Wang C, Yu H, Horby PW, *et al.* Comparison of patients hospitalized with influenza A subtypes H7N9, H5N1, and 2009 pandemic H1N1. *Clin Infect Dis* 2014; 58: 1095–1103.
102. Yu H, Gao Z, Feng Z, *et al.* Clinical characteristics of 26 human cases of highly pathogenic avian influenza A (H5N1) virus infection in China. *PLoS One* 2008; 3: e2985.
103. Mertz D, Kim TH, Johnstone J, *et al.* Populations at risk for severe or complicated Avian Influenza H5N1: a systematic review and meta-analysis. *PLoS One* 2014; 9: e89697.
104. Dugas AF, Valsamakis A, Atreya MR, *et al.* Clinical diagnosis of influenza in the ED. *Am J Emerg Med* 2015; 33: 770–775.
105. Gharabaghi F, Hawan A, Drews SJ, *et al.* Evaluation of multiple commercial molecular and conventional diagnostic assays for the detection of respiratory viruses in children. *Clin Microbiol Infect* 2011; 17: 1900–1906.
106. Caliendo AM. Multiplex PCR and emerging technologies for the detection of respiratory pathogens. *Clin Infect Dis* 2011; 52: Suppl. 4, S326–S330.
107. Zhong NS, Li YM, Yang ZF, *et al.* Chinese guidelines for diagnosis and treatment of influenza (2011). *J Thorac Dis* 2011; 3: 274–289.
108. World Health Organization. Interim WHO surveillance recommendations for human infection with avian influenza A(H7N9) virus. www.who.int/influenza/human_animal_interface/influenza_h7n9/InterimSurveillanceRecH7N9_10May13.pdf?ua=1 Data last accessed: March 16, 2016. Data last updated: May 10, 2013.
109. Chen Y, Liang W, Yang S, *et al.* Human infections with the emerging avian influenza A H7N9 virus from wet market poultry: clinical analysis and characterisation of viral genome. *Lancet* 2013; 381: 1916–1925.
110. Nguyen HT, Nguyen T, Mishin VP, *et al.* Antiviral susceptibility of highly pathogenic avian influenza A(H5N1) viruses isolated from poultry, Vietnam, 2009–2011. *Emerg Infect Dis* 2013; 19: 1963–1971.
111. Hurt AC, Selleck P, Komadina N, *et al.* Susceptibility of highly pathogenic A(H5N1) avian influenza viruses to the neuraminidase inhibitors and adamantanes. *Antiviral Res* 2007; 73: 228–231.

112. Muthuri SG, Venkatesan S, Myles PR, *et al.* Effectiveness of neuraminidase inhibitors in reducing mortality in patients admitted to hospital with influenza A H1N1pdm09 virus infection: a meta-analysis of individual participant data. *Lancet Respir Med* 2014; 2: 395–404.
113. Yang SG, Cao B, Liang LR, *et al.* Antiviral therapy and outcomes of patients with pneumonia caused by influenza A pandemic (H1N1) virus. *PLoS One* 2012; 7: e29652.
114. Ng S, Cowling BJ, Fang VJ, *et al.* Effects of oseltamivir treatment on duration of clinical illness and viral shedding and household transmission of influenza virus. *Clin Infect Dis* 2010; 50: 707–714.
115. Cheung DH, Tsang TK, Fang VJ, *et al.* Association of oseltamivir treatment with virus shedding, illness, and household transmission of influenza viruses. *J Infect Dis* 2015; 212: 391–396.
116. Fry AM, Goswami D, Nahar K, *et al.* Efficacy of oseltamivir treatment started within 5 days of symptom onset to reduce influenza illness duration and virus shedding in an urban setting in Bangladesh: a randomised placebo-controlled trial. *Lancet Infect Dis* 2014; 14: 109–118.
117. World Health Organization. WHO guidelines for pharmacological management of pandemic (H1N1) 2009 influenza and other influenza viruses. www.who.int/csr/resources/publications/swineflu/h1n1_use_antivirals_20090820/en/ Date last accessed: March 16, 2016. Date last updated: February 10, 2010.
118. Fairchok MP, Chen WJ, Arnold JC, *et al.* Neuraminidase inhibitor therapy in a military population. *J Clin Virol* 2015; 67: 17–22.
119. Le QM, Kiso M, Someya K, *et al.* Avian flu: isolation of drug-resistant H5N1 virus. *Nature* 2005; 437: 1108.
120. Memoli MJ, Athota R, Reed S, *et al.* The natural history of influenza infection in the severely immunocompromised *vs* nonimmunocompromised hosts. *Clin Infect Dis* 2014; 58: 214–224.
121. Lee N, Leo YS, Cao B, *et al.* Neuraminidase inhibitors, superinfection and corticosteroids affect survival of influenza patients. *Eur Respir J* 2015; 45: 1642–1652.
122. Adisasmito W, Chan PK, Lee N, *et al.* Effectiveness of antiviral treatment in human influenza A(H5N1) infections: analysis of a Global Patient Registry. *J Infect Dis* 2010; 202: 1154–1160.
123. Chan PK, Lee N, Zaman M, *et al.* Determinants of antiviral effectiveness in influenza virus A subtype H5N1. *J Infect Dis* 2012; 206: 1359–1366.
124. South East Asia Infectious Disease Clinical Research Network. Effect of double dose oseltamivir on clinical and virological outcomes in children and adults admitted to hospital with severe influenza: double blind randomised controlled trial. *BMJ* 2013; 346: f3039.
125. Fiore AE, Fry A, Shay D, *et al.* Antiviral agents for the treatment and chemoprophylaxis of influenza – recommendations of the Advisory Committee on Immunization Practices (ACIP). *MMWR Recomm Rep* 2011; 60: 1–24.
126. To KK, Chan JF, Yuen KY. Viral lung infections: epidemiology, virology, clinical features, and management of avian influenza A(H7N9). *Curr Opin Pulm Med* 2014; 20: 225–232.
127. Li TC, Chan MC, Lee N. Clinical implications of antiviral resistance in influenza. *Viruses* 2015; 7: 4929–4944.
128. Dunning J, Baillie JK, Cao B, *et al.* Antiviral combinations for severe influenza. *Lancet Infect Dis* 2014; 14: 1259–1270.
129. Kim SH, Hong SB, Yun SC, *et al.* Corticosteroid treatment in critically ill patients with pandemic influenza A/H1N1 2009 infection: analytic strategy using propensity scores. *Am J Respir Crit Care Med* 2011; 183: 1207–1214.
130. Brun-Buisson C, Richard JC, Mercat A, *et al.* Early corticosteroids in severe influenza A/H1N1 pneumonia and acute respiratory distress syndrome. *Am J Respir Crit Care Med* 2011; 183: 1200–1206.
131. Rodrigo C, Leonardi-Bee J, Nguyen-Van-Tam JS, *et al.* Effect of corticosteroid therapy on influenza-related mortality: a systematic review and meta-analysis. *J Infect Dis* 2015; 212: 183–194.
132. Cao B, Gao H, Zhou B, *et al.* Adjuvant corticosteroid treatment in adults with influenza A (H7N9) viral pneumonia. *Crit Care Med* 2016 [In press; DOI: 10.1097/ccm.0000000000001616].
133. Cao B, Hayden FG. Therapy of H7N9 pneumonia: current perspectives. *Expert Rev Anti Infect Ther* 2013; 11: 1123–1126.
134. Dellinger RP, Levy MM, Rhodes A, *et al.* Surviving sepsis campaign: international guidelines for management of severe sepsis and septic shock: 2012. *Crit Care Med* 2013; 41: 580–637.
135. Brundage JF. Interactions between influenza and bacterial respiratory pathogens: implications for pandemic preparedness. *Lancet Infect Dis* 2006; 6: 303–312.
136. Chertow DS, Memoli MJ. Bacterial coinfection in influenza: a grand rounds review. *JAMA* 2013; 309: 275–282.
137. Madhi SA, Cutland CL, Kuwanda L, *et al.* Influenza vaccination of pregnant women and protection of their infants. *N Engl J Med* 2014; 371: 918–931.
138. Darvishian M, Bijlsma MJ, Hak E, *et al.* Effectiveness of seasonal influenza vaccine in community-dwelling elderly people: a meta-analysis of test-negative design case-control studies. *Lancet Infect Dis* 2014; 14: 1228–1239.
139. Thompson MG, Li DK, Shifflett P, *et al.* Effectiveness of seasonal trivalent influenza vaccine for preventing influenza virus illness among pregnant women: a population-based case-control study during the 2010–2011 and 2011–2012 influenza seasons. *Clin Infect Dis* 2014; 58: 449–457.
140. Grijalva CG, Zhu Y, Williams DJ, *et al.* Association between hospitalization with community-acquired laboratory-confirmed influenza pneumonia and prior receipt of influenza vaccination. *JAMA* 2015; 314: 1488–1497.

141. Leroux-Roels G. Prepandemic H5N1 influenza vaccine adjuvanted with AS03: a review of the pre-clinical and clinical data. *Expert Opin Biol Ther* 2009; 9: 1057–1071.
142. Kosalaraksa P, Jeanfreau R, Frenette L, *et al.* AS03B-adjuvanted H5N1 influenza vaccine in children 6 months through 17 years of age: a phase 2/3 randomized, placebo-controlled, observer-blinded trial. *J Infect Dis* 2015; 211: 801–810.
143. Yu H, Wu JT, Cowling BJ, *et al.* Effect of closure of live poultry markets on poultry-to-person transmission of avian influenza A H7N9 virus: an ecological study. *Lancet* 2014; 383: 541–548.
144. Fournié G, Guitian FJ, Mangtani P, *et al.* Impact of the implementation of rest days in live bird markets on the dynamics of H5N1 highly pathogenic avian influenza. *J R Soc Interface* 2011; 8: 1079–1089.
145. Kung NY, Guan Y, Perkins NR, *et al.* The impact of a monthly rest day on avian influenza virus isolation rates in retail live poultry markets in Hong Kong. *Avian Dis* 2003; 47: 1037–1041.
146. Yee KS, Carpenter TE, Mize S, *et al.* The live bird market system and low-pathogenic avian influenza prevention in southern California. *Avian Dis* 2008; 52: 348–352.

Disclosures: B. Cao was funded by the National Science Grant for Distinguished Young Scholars (grant number: 81425001/H0104) and the National Key Technology Support Program from the Ministry of Science and Technology (grant number: 2015BAI12B00).

Chapter 5

Respiratory syncytial virus

Akhilesh Jha, Hannah Jarvis, Clementine Fraser and Peter J.M. Openshaw

RSV infection has an estimated global incidence of 33 million cases in children <5 years of age, with 10% requiring hospital admission and up to 199000 dying of the disease. There is growing evidence that severe infantile RSV bronchiolitis, a condition characterised by an inflammatory reaction to the virus, is associated with later childhood wheeze in some vulnerable children; however, a direct causal relationship with asthma has not yet been established. RSV infection is also increasingly recognised as a cause of morbidity and mortality in those with underlying airway disease, the immunocompromised and frail elderly persons. Novel molecular-based diagnostic tools are becoming established, but treatment remains largely supportive, with palivizumab the only licensed agent currently available for passive prophylaxis of selected pre-term infants. While effective treatments remain elusive, there is optimism about the testing of novel antiviral drugs and the development of vaccines that may induce long-lasting immunity without the risk of disease augmentation.

Since its discovery in 1956, RSV has become recognised as a leading global cause of morbidity and mortality, especially among infants in the first 6 months of life. RSV is the commonest cause of childhood ARI and is the major single cause of hospitalisation during infancy. In recent decades, it has been realised that RSV also afflicts various at-risk adults, including the frail elderly and immunocompromised persons. In resource-poor settings, it is an important cause of death due to due to lower respiratory tract infection, second only to pneumococcal pneumonia and *Haemophilus influenzae* type B. Resource-limited countries have more than twice the incidence of severe disease seen in developed countries and, remarkably, 99% of the global deaths caused by RSV infection [1].

Given this appalling disease toll and the fact that current treatment is simply supportive, it is clear that prevention, early diagnosis and the discovery of specific therapies have enormous potential to improve global health among the most vulnerable in society. RSV remains one of the last major viruses for which we currently (in early 2016) have no safe and effective vaccine.

Not only does RSV cause acute disease, but those with severe infections can be left with long-term sequelae. These include persistent wheeze and, in some cases, established inflammatory airway disease [2, 3], highlighting the importance of understanding which immune responses correlate with protection and what makes some individuals at risk of

Respiratory Sciences, National Heart and Lung Institute, Imperial College London (St Mary's Campus), London, UK.

Correspondence: Peter J.M. Openshaw, National Heart and Lung Institute, Imperial College London (St Mary's Campus), Norfolk Place, Paddington, London, W2 1PG, UK. E-mail: p.openshaw@imperial.ac.uk

 Print ISBN: 978-1-84984-069-9. Online ISBN: 978-1-84984-070-5. Print ISSN: 2312-508X. Online ISSN: 2312-5098.

severe or delayed disease. Molecular techniques such as real-time PCR have become more affordable, and offer rapid and accurate diagnosis, with the ability to identify the disease earlier in at-risk patients at levels of viral burden too low for conventional detection, affording the potential for community-based epidemiology [4, 5]. Intensive research in recent decades has accelerated progress on many fronts, with several promising new vaccines in advanced stages of development [6, 7]. In countries with limited access to healthcare, an effective and affordable vaccine would be transformative.

Epidemiology

RSV causes significant morbidity and mortality across the world and is the leading cause of pneumonia and bronchiolitis in infants. In addition to a currently poorly quantified burden in the elderly, it is estimated to cause 30 million ARIs and more than 60 000 childhood deaths worldwide each year [1, 8]. The main burden of disease is in the under 5 years age group, but RSV also has considerable impact on various at-risk adult populations [9, 10]. In the USA, RSV is estimated to cause 17 358 deaths per year, 22% of which occur in persons <65 years of age [11].

Seasonality

The seasonality of RSV infection varies across the world. Temperate zones tend to experience RSV epidemics during late autumn, winter and/or spring [12], whereas tropical and arctic climates see less well-defined annual variation, with year-round disease described in some settings [13]. In northern tropical areas, seasonality is associated with a decrease in temperature and an increase in rainfall, whereas in more tropical climates yearly outbreaks can occur during the warm and rainy seasons (figure 1) [14, 15].

In Europe, RSV is predominantly a disease of winter, with peaks of illness in December and January in the UK, Belgium, Germany and the Netherlands, with a later peak in March in Mediterranean countries, such as Greece [16, 17]; biennial cycles of RSV activity have been described in northern Europe [15]. The association of an increase in RSV cases with declining temperatures has been attributed to: 1) increased indoor crowding, leading to enhanced viral transmission; 2) lower temperatures increasing viral stability; 3) chilling of the host, increasing host susceptibility; and 4) lower temperatures or host chilling, increasing activation of dormant virus [18].

Infants and children

Pneumonia is the leading cause of mortality in children worldwide, with RSV being the commonest single cause of ARI in young children [8, 19]. By 18 months of age, 87% of children have antibodies to RSV, and by the age of 3 years, virtually all children have been infected [20].

A large meta-analysis estimated there to be 33.8 million cases of RSV-associated ARI worldwide in 2005 in children <5 years of age, but this is likely to be an underestimate; previous studies using active methods for data collection, such as home visits, have shown much higher incidence rates [1]. In the USA, RSV has been estimated to account for 20% of ARI hospitalisations in children under 5 years (17 per 1000 children <6 months of age and 3 per 1000 children under 5 years of age), but 99% of RSV deaths occur in low-income countries, with a lack of access to basic supportive care being a key factor [1, 8]. Children are at highest risk of death in the first 6 months of life [11].

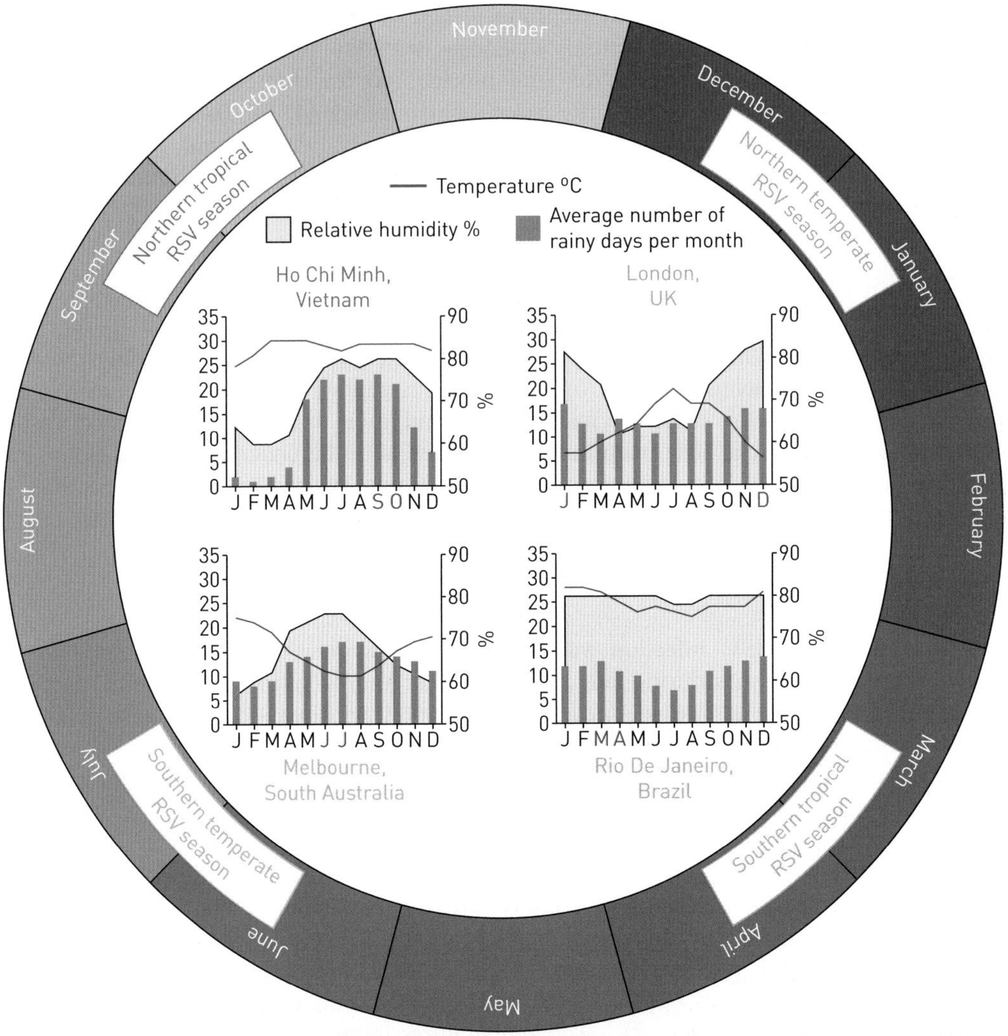

Figure 1. Annual cycle of global peak RSV incidence and associated climactic factors. Temperate countries typically have peak incidence of RSV during their winter months, which are associated with lower temperatures, higher rainfall and higher humidity. There is greater variability in tropical regions, which are prone to biennial and perennial RSV. Limited information is available for some regions, *e.g.* Africa. Data from [12–15].

The majority of children suffering from RSV-associated ARI have no underlying comorbidities. Low birth weight and prematurity are major risk factors for hospitalisation, as is congenital or acquired immunodeficiency and various cardiopulmonary, chronic lung disease and neurodevelopmental disorders [21, 22]. Environmental factors contributing to increased susceptibility are side-stream tobacco smoke exposure, lack of breastfeeding and low socioeconomic status [23].

Adults and elderly persons

There is still no globally accepted definition or reliable classification of ARI, making it difficult to compare studies and to make accurate estimates of disease burden. Adding to these problems, variations in sampling methodology and diagnostic testing across studies provide further hurdles. With major differences in healthcare provision and access to resources in different geographical and socioeconomic settings, it is difficult to estimate the true impact of RSV disease in diverse settings. Despite these caveats, we can state with reasonable certainty that it is rare for healthy immunocompetent adults to require hospitalisation due to RSV infection.

However, infection with RSV is so prevalent that it is estimated to cause a disease burden at least comparable to influenza in elderly persons [24]. Given the ageing population structure in Western countries, adult RSV-associated mortality is becoming an ever-greater problem that poses a huge health and economic burden [9, 11]. A recent North American study examined the impact of RSV during four consecutive winters among healthy elderly patients (n=608), high-risk adults (those with chronic heart or lung disease, n=540) and patients hospitalised with acute respiratory illness (n=1388). The average age across all groups was >70 years; RSV infection developed annually in 3–7% of healthy elderly patients and in 4–10% of high-risk adults, and was present in 8–13% of patients hospitalised with ARI. During the study period, RSV infection accounted for 11% of hospitalisations for pneumonia, 11% for COPD, 5% for congestive heart failure and 7% for asthma [10]. In the UK, it is estimated that, among the adult population, those over >65 years of age account for 36% of general practice episodes, 79% of hospitalisations and 93% of deaths due to RSV each season, and that RSV is responsible for more morbidity than influenza [24]. Globally, RSV accounts for 7.4% of elderly (>65 years) individuals presenting with ILI [25].

The immunocompromised

In both children and adults, various immunodeficiency states predispose to RSV infection and disease. In addition to HIV-infected children being liable to develop RSV-associated ARI, they are 3.5 times more likely to be hospitalised than non-HIV-infected children [21], are more likely to present with pneumonia, have greater evidence of bacterial coinfection and have higher mortality rates than non-HIV-infected children [26]. RSV is a common cause of ARI in haematopoietic stem cell transplant patients, with rates of infection being as high as 2–17% in some settings [27]. As well as increased susceptibility to infection, these patients are also liable to progress to more severe disease [27]. RSV pneumonia in this patient group has a mortality of up to 83% [27]. Factors linked to severity and poor outcome include male sex, the type of graft (allogeneic), the myeloablative regimen, CMV seropositivity, increasing age, an unrelated donor transplant, graft-*versus*-host disease and becoming infected within the first 3 months of transplant [28].

Virology

RSV is an enveloped virus belonging to the genus *Pneumovirus*, family *Paramyxoviridae*. It is a negative-sense, single-stranded RNA virus consisting of 11 proteins encoded within a 15.2 kb genome. It has a non-segmented genome so, unlike influenza, it does not have the capacity for reassortment of genome segments leading to antigenic shifts with the potential to cause large pandemics.

RSV was originally characterised in 1956 from a colony of chimpanzees with coryza and was termed chimpanzee coryza agent [29]. It was later isolated from a number of infants and was recognised as a human virus that caused mild illness in a susceptible group of chimpanzees [30]. It was renamed RSV, as it causes infected cells to fuse with neighbouring cells, creating large multinucleated syncytia.

RSV has been classified into two distinct subgroups (A and B), based on antigenic variability [31]. These two groups have been described based on the reactions of two major surface proteins to monoclonal antibodies (mAbs): the glycoprotein (G) facilitates viral attachment to host ciliated cells of the airway [32], while the fusion (F) protein mediates virion and host cell fusion [33].

Additional antigenic variability occurs within the A and B subgroups, with the most extensive antigenic and genetic diversity being found in the G protein, which therefore plays a significant role in RSV pathogenicity and immune evasion. Subtype A RSV may be marginally more virulent and may replicate to higher titres than the group B viruses *in vivo* and *in vitro* [34]. New RSV genotypes appear periodically and tend to predominate and replace the circulating strain of RSV. However, the original circulating strain does not become extinct, with new and old genotypes occurring alongside each other for relatively long periods [35].

Viral structure and proteins

RSV particles are pleomorphic, with both spherical and filamentous particles of different sizes [36]. The virions display three surface proteins: F, G and SH (small hydrophobic) (figure 2) [37]. The G and F proteins are integral for virion attachment and fusion, binding to disaccharide subunits called glycosaminoglycans and RhoA, respectively [38, 39]. Following fusion, the virion releases the nucleocapsid into the cytosol, enabling the RNA to enter the host cell. The M2 mRNA has two overlapping ORFs encoding M2-1 and M2-2. The M2-2 protein governs the transition from transcription to production of genomic RNA [40]. The large (L) protein is a viral RNA-dependent RNA polymerase that carries out multiple enzyme functions required for RSV replication. mRNA is transcribed from the genomic RNA, generating a complete positive-sense RNA complement of the genome, called the antigenome, which acts as a template for replication. Throughout replication, the nucleoprotein (N) encapsulates the RNA, preventing its degradation. The matrix (M) protein co-ordinates the assembly of the envelope proteins with the nucleocapsid proteins (N, phosphoprotein (P) and M2-1), and facilitates budding of new immature virions using the host cell membrane. Filamentous virions show a helical assembly of M proteins, which play a critical role in the formation of infectious filamentous particles [41].

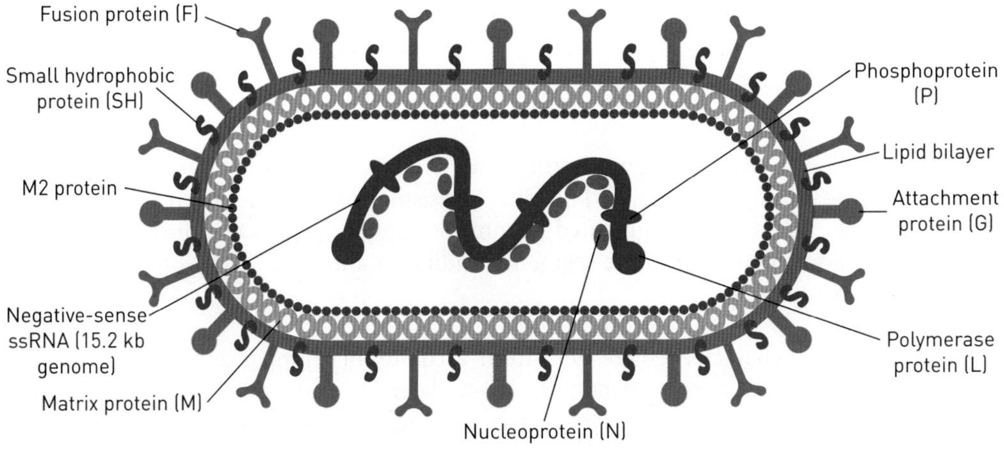

Figure 2. Diagrammatic cross-section through an infectious RSV filament. ss: single-stranded.

Pathogenesis

RSV is a highly contagious virus and can cause outbreaks in both community and hospital settings [42, 43]. Infection begins by inoculation of the nose or eyes *via* large-particles aerosols or direct contact with an infected person, with an incubation period of 2–8 days. RSV can survive for prolonged periods on skin, cloth and other objects, facilitating its spread [44]. How it survives so well is puzzling, as laboratory-grown virus is notoriously unstable at room temperature [45].

RSV infects the ciliated epithelial cells of the upper and lower respiratory tracts. In the lower airways, the virus specifically targets the ciliated cells of the bronchioles, but can also be found in type 1 pneumocytes and intraepithelial dendritic cells. More recently, it has been demonstrated that RSV can infect basal cells (the progenitors for the conducting airway epithelium), where it has the potential to influence the morphogenesis of the airway epithelium [46].

Infection causes widespread inflammation with peribronchial monocyte and T-cell infiltration, epithelial necrosis, submucosal oedema and mucus overproduction [47]. Infection and tissue damage tends to be patchy rather than diffuse. Airway obstruction occurs in the small airways, secondary to sloughing of epithelial cells, mucus plugs, and accumulated luminal and intraluminal immune cells. Additionally, syncytia are occasionally observed, more commonly in immunocompromised patients [48]. The degree to which this depends on viral or host variation is currently poorly understood. Possibly, the development of severe disease results from an unfortunate collision of a particular viral strain with a host that responds adversely to that specific strain.

Environmental factors

Environmental factors include exposure to tobacco smoke, air pollution and indoor crowding (day-care attendance, nursing home or hospital stay). The presence of an older sibling is an independent risk factor for the development of RSV disease in infancy [16]. There have been many studies that have documented the link between tobacco smoke and RSV infection. A 2012 systematic review of 30 studies reported that tobacco smoke exposure placed infants and young children at increased risk of hospitalisation for RSV-attributable lower respiratory tract infection, in addition to increasing the severity of illness [49]. The association between air pollution and severe RSV disease is also well documented; for example, has been shown *in vivo* that diesel engine emissions cause a more pronounced peribronchial/bronchiolar inflammation, with increased mucous cell metaplasia, in the context of RSV infection [50].

Viral factors

There is a well-documented correlation between the level of virus replication and the severity of infection [51, 52]. Unlike other viruses, immunity to RSV infection is incomplete and short lived, and re-infection is common throughout life. This is not largely attributable to viral evolution in response to host immunity; instead, RSV seems to be able to modulate and evade the immune system. It does this in several ways. The G protein is key to this, being present in membrane-bound and secreted forms. Secretory G protein acts as a decoy, aiding virus evasion of antibody-mediated neutralisation [53]. It also exhibits a CX3C fractalkine-like motif, which binds to the chemokine receptor CX3CR1, inducing leucocyte chemotaxis [54]. Additionally, the cysteine-rich portion of the G protein is able to directly inhibit signalling from TLR2, -4 and -9, all of which reduce the host immune response.

Furthermore, two nonstructural (NS) proteins, NS1 and NS2, which are highly expressed during early RSV infection, downregulate IFN production and apoptosis, leading to enhanced viral replication [55]. The SH transmembrane protein increases membrane permeability, and to a lesser extent has also been linked to decreased apoptosis [56]. Within the virion, the RNA is tightly bound by N protein, and this is thought to prevent degradation and also to aid with concealment from pattern-recognition receptors, promoting infectivity in host cells.

Host factors

Multiple factors can increase susceptibility to RSV infection and are associated with a more severe disease course. These include premature birth, comorbidities (cardiac and respiratory), immunodeficiency and age. There is increasing evidence that there may be some genetic associations of RSV susceptibility and severity. For example, it has been shown that identical twins are often concordant for severe RSV disease. The host genetic contribution for this propensity is estimated to account for approximately 20% of the variance [57].

The genetic polymorphisms that affect RSV pathogenesis often lie in genes involved in innate defences, surfactant proteins, host cell receptors, neutrophil responses, T-helper cell (Th)1 and Th2 responses, and other components of adaptive immunity [58]. Ongoing genome-wide approaches are likely to further improve our knowledge in this area.

Immune response

As described above, virtually all children are infected by the age of 2 years; most immunocompetent children clear the infection within 3 weeks [59]. Some infants are predisposed to more severe infection, and those infected in the first 6 months of life are subsequently prone to wheeze until at least 6 years of age [3], and possibly through to adulthood [2].

Early immune responses

The recognition of pathogen-associated molecular patterns, knowns as PAMPs, present on viruses by pattern-recognition receptors, such as TLRs and RNA-sensing RIG-I-like receptors, leads to the release of antimicrobial mediators by the host mucosal immune system and serves to form an effective first line of resistance against infection. Type 1 responses are characterised by the release of type I IFNs (IFN-α and IFN-β) and type III IFNs (IFN-λ1, IFN-λ2 and IFN-λ3) [60]. These are potent antiviral mediators induced early in infection from epithelial cells and resident immune cells, with alveolar macrophages recently being discovered in a murine model to be major contributors to IFN production leading to the subsequent recruitment of inflammatory monocytes to the lungs [61]. Dendritic cells are also key to bridging innate and adaptive responses by transporting viral antigens to the cervical and pulmonary lymph nodes and presenting them to $CD4^+$ T-lymphocytes, which in turn activates $CD8^+$ T- and B-lymphocytes. They return to the site of infection to further promote local induction of pro-inflammatory mediators and cellular efflux [62].

There is debate about whether defective or exuberant immune responses are responsible for the infection spreading from a limited mucosal infection (in most people) to more extensive lung immunopathology or even extrapulmonary manifestations (in susceptible individuals) [63–65]. An insufficient type 1 response as well as exaggerated type 2 responses (characterised by IL-4, IL-5 and IL-13) have been implicated in causing susceptibility to RSV bronchiolitis [66, 67], and an inability to produce sufficient IFN-γ early in life may increase the risk of developing severe disease [68]. Gene polymorphisms of TLR4, IL-4 receptor α and IL-8 have also been associated with severe RSV bronchiolitis, highlighting the important role of innate immunity, although their biological role in active disease is yet to be fully understood [69–71].

The naïve immune system of infants is characterised by hyporesponsiveness to infections and viral mimetic stimuli *in vitro* when compared with that of adults [64, 72], with premature infants of <35 weeks' gestational age being at highest risk due to compromised pulmonary development and deficient serum immunoglobulins [73]. In term infants, maternal-specific RSV-neutralising antibodies are present from the third trimester and are stable until birth, with higher cord blood levels being protective against RSV infection, although only for the first 6 months of life [74].

Established infection, re-infection and resolution

Once infection is established, cellular immunity and immunoregulation play a critical role in promoting viral clearance and limiting pathology, which is clearly demonstrated in paediatric patients with primary or acquired immunodeficiency, who have a much longer duration of infection and can shed virus for several months [75, 76]. Classically, Th1 cells, which make IFN-γ, are important in antiviral defence, but it is possible that other Th cell subsets contribute towards eliminating the virus [77]. In particular, IL-10-producing cells inhibit disease and inflammation in mice infected with RSV, especially during recovery [78]. Cytotoxic $CD8^+$ T-lymphocytes may cause neutrophil efflux [79, 80], while more abundant airway-resident memory T-cells at baseline correlate with reduced viral load and symptoms during experimental human adult infection [81]. Interestingly, both virus and T-cell inflammation may remain present in asymptomatic convalescent volunteers in this model [81]. Certain macrophage subtypes (M2) and plasmacytoid dendritic cells probably play an important role in modulating local immune responses and restricting T-cell-mediated inflammation [82, 83]. The ability of RSV to re-infect may also be explained by defective RSV-specific IgA memory B-cell responses [84, 85]. Some individuals suffer dual infection with RSV and other viruses, which can lead to greater severity of disease and is associated with decreased IFN-γ responses [86].

It is thought that the increased susceptibility and severity of RSV in the elderly is secondary to immunosenescence, but how this occurs has not been fully defined. It has been shown that elderly and younger individuals have comparable RSV neutralisation antibody titres but that there may be an impairment of T-cell-mediated immunity [87, 88]. Studies of RSV disease in mice have indicated the importance of regulatory T-cells in maintaining an effective and nonpathogenic response to RSV infection, and have highlighted the dysregulation of immune responses that are characteristic of bronchiolitis [89].

Clinical manifestations

Acute presentation in children

RSV infection in children can result in a range of disease phenotypes from mild upper respiratory tract symptoms to life-threatening lower airway involvement necessitating hospital admission and mechanical ventilation. Infants are at greater risk from RSV infection than older children, with an increased likelihood of lower airway involvement in the form of both bronchiolitis and pneumonia [1].

Clinical presentation of RSV often begins with typical upper respiratory tract signs and symptoms, including coryza, cough and febrile illness [90]. On examination, rhinitis and pharyngitis may be seen in association with conjunctival signs and erythema to the tympanic membrane [64]. Less frequently, bulging of the tympanic membrane may be seen if otitis media is also present [64]. Nasal congestion and generalised malaise can lead to poor feeding, and subsequently dehydration [64].

In approximately one-third of infants with viral respiratory infections, progression to lower respiratory tract involvement is observed [64], most commonly in the form of bronchiolitis, although pneumonia and laryngotracheitis (croup) can also develop [91]. Bronchiolitis presents as worsening respiratory function with tachypnoea, wheeze and noisy breathing, as well as systemic viral features, such as fever and lethargy [90, 91]. Some infants develop vomiting and poor feeding with dehydration [64]. In young infants, apnoea has also been described [92], and indeed may be the presenting symptom early in the disease. Signs of respiratory distress, including nasal flaring, costal and intercostal recession, and cyanosis, should be assessed by clinicians when determining the need for admission to hospital, in addition to other markers of disease severity, including hydration status and level of alertness. Polyphonic expiratory wheeze and fine crepitations may be heard on auscultation of the chest [91]. According to current guidelines, chest radiographs are not performed routinely in children with simple bronchiolitis but may show features of hyperexpansion, including increased anterior–posterior diameter and diaphragmatic flattening, as well as patchy bilateral infiltrates and atelectasis (figure 3) [90, 93]. Pneumonia with consolidation seen on chest radiography may be due to the virus itself or to a secondary bacterial infection.

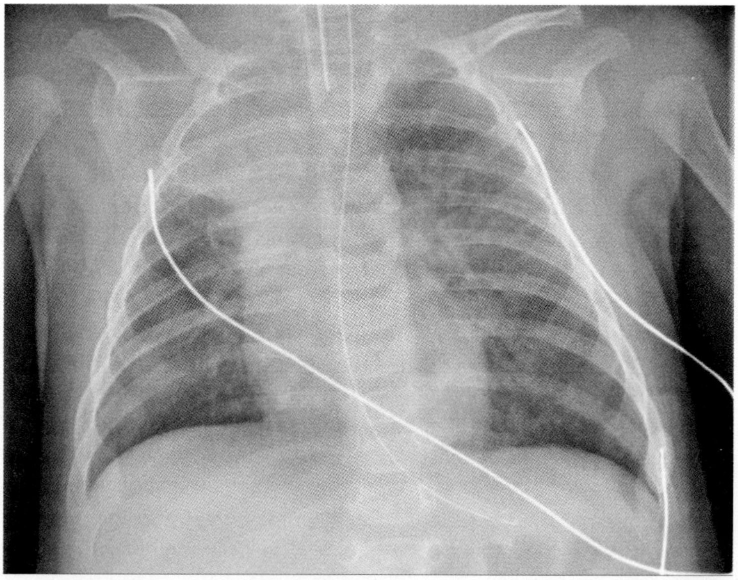

Figure 3. Chest radiograph of a 3-month-old infant with severe RSV bronchiolitis, demonstrating a collapsed right upper lobe, hyperinflated left lung and bilateral perihilar, peribronchial thickening. The patient is intubated and has a nasogastric tube *in situ*.

Extrapulmonary manifestations of RSV are uncommon but have been described, and include seizures, hyponatraemia, cardiac arrhythmia and failure, and hepatitis [65].

The differential diagnosis for children presenting with signs and symptoms of lower and upper respiratory infection includes other viral infections, such as rhinovirus, metapneumovirus and influenza virus; primary bacterial pneumonia; congenital conditions, such as cystic fibrosis; asthma; and inhaled foreign bodies.

Longer-term complications in children

In addition to the significant health burden of acute RSV infection, there is evidence of longer-term consequences to respiratory function, with the development of persistent airway disease. Although a causal relationship remains unclear, an association between RSV infection as an infant and subsequent wheezing, allergy and asthma, sometimes persisting into adulthood, has been demonstrated [2, 90, 94].

Several longitudinal cohort studies have tracked the incidence of respiratory illness in children with RSV infection in infancy. The Tucson Children's Respiratory Study (TCRS) examined outcomes in children with clinician-confirmed RSV lower respiratory tract infection (defined by the presence of cough, wheeze, breathlessness, hoarseness or stridor, in the presence of an RSV-positive diagnostic test) contracted up to 3 years of age. They reported an increased prevalence of wheeze in these children up to 11 years and persistently impaired lung function until 13 years of age [95]. Sigurs *et al.* [2] investigated a more severely affected group of children who had been hospitalised with RSV lower respiratory tract infection in the first year of life. Their findings correlated with those seen in the less severely affected children, with an increased prevalence of asthma/recurrent wheeze, as well as atopy and clinical allergy, which persisted throughout childhood [2]. The data collected from these participants at 18 years of age continued to show differences between healthy controls and affected individuals in the relative rates of allergy, asthma and recurrent wheeze, as well as abnormalities in lung function [2]. They postulated that persistent clinical and lung function abnormalities represent the consequences of airway remodelling stimulated by early RSV infection [2]. The potential pathogenic mechanisms for this remain unclear, although impaired T-regulatory cell function, persistent activation of innate immunity and an early Th2 switch have been implicated [96].

Debate remains as to the extent to which early RSV infection causes later airway disease by altering immune responses and subsequent airway maturation, or whether children with a predisposition to wheeze and asthma are more likely to develop severe RSV infection. To address this question, a double-blind placebo-controlled trial was designed to investigate whether prevention of RSV, using the mAb palivizumab during RSV season, would impact on subsequent rates of wheeze [97]. The results demonstrated a substantial reduction in episodes of wheeze for up to 1 year in healthy pre-term babies in the treatment group compared with those in the placebo group [97]. Of note, the effect of palivizumab on wheeze reduction persisted, even after treatment had been stopped and the RSV season was complete, suggesting that wheeze reduction was not simply attributable to fewer acute RSV episodes [97]. The authors argued that their findings support the concept of RSV as a pathogenic stimulus in the development of recurrent wheeze. They postulated that epithelial damage from RSV infection alters local pulmonary immune responses, resulting in airway hyperresponsiveness [97]. However, testing of a high-potency derivative of palivizumab (motavizumab) showed no such effect in term babies, despite a substantial reduction in hospital admissions and noninferiority compared with palivizumab [98, 99]. The reasons for the disparity between these two mAb drugs are unclear, and may simply be evidence against a direct causal relationship between RSV and subsequent wheeze. Another possible explanation lies in the differences between the study populations: the palivizumab study investigated outcomes in pre-term babies and was based on parent-reported episodes of wheeze, whereas the motavizumab study examined healthy term infants and relied on medically attended wheezing episodes [99].

Presentation in adults

For the majority of adults infected with RSV, the extent of symptoms is minimal, with nonspecific features of a viral upper respiratory tract infection including coryza, sore throat, fever and malaise, as well as lower respiratory tract symptoms, such as cough [100]. Those with underlying immune compromise or cardiorespiratory disease, or the elderly, may experience significantly more morbidity and mortality [9, 10]. The presentation of RSV in elderly patients is similar to that seen in younger adults, although with a greater severity and increased likelihood of lower respiratory tract involvement [100]. Typically, RSV illness begins with nasal congestion before progressing to cough in 90–97% of patients [9, 101]. Compared with influenza, systemic symptoms, including fever, myalgia and gastrointestinal complaints, are less common [102]. In contrast to other respiratory tract viral infections, wheeze is frequently noted, even in those without underlying airway disease. Audible crackles on chest examination and infiltrates on chest radiography occur in 30–50% of elderly patients [9].

In addition to these common respiratory symptoms, immunocompromised patients are predisposed to otalgia, and clinical or radiological evidence of sinusitis in these individuals can be useful in distinguishing RSV from other viral causes of infection, including CMV [100, 103]. Chest radiographs in these patients are frequently abnormal, ranging from interstitial infiltrates to alveolar shadowing and pleural effusions. The severity of infection is closely linked to the degree of immune compromise, with bone marrow transplant recipients being at greatest risk. Such patients have pneumonia rates of up to 79% and mortality of 78% post-transplant following infection with RSV [104].

RSV can also cause a deterioration of underlying cardiorespiratory disease. Estimating the percentage of acute exacerbations of COPD attributable to RSV infection is difficult, as the appropriate viral diagnostic tests are not employed routinely in clinical practice, but estimates range up 22% [105]. While asthma exacerbations are triggered primarily by rhinovirus, RSV and influenza infection are important contributors to morbidity [106, 107]. In patients with lung transplants, infection with RSV can result in an acute pneumonitis presenting with increasing breathlessness, cough, wheeze and a decrease in lung function [108].

As with children, longer-term complications can be seen in adults following recovery from acute RSV infection. In patients with COPD, a permanent decline in lung function following clinical recovery from an exacerbation is well documented [109]. Likewise, in lung transplant recipients, RSV infection has been implicated in the development of chronic graft dysfunction characterised by obliterative bronchiolitis [110], with small airway remodelling and air trapping. Evidence for the persistence of RSV infection with the development of a latent state has been reported in a variety of animal models and in observational human studies [111]. Although not all studies have supported this hypothesis

[112], the potential impact of persistent infection, not only as a reservoir for ongoing viral transmission but also in perpetuating pulmonary immunopathology, could be significant.

Laboratory diagnosis

The American Academy of Pediatrics (AAP) does not recommend routine use of laboratory techniques to diagnose RSV bronchiolitis, which should be based primarily on clinical assessment [113]. However, due to the many acute viral and bacterial respiratory infections that cause symptoms similar to RSV, an accurate laboratory diagnosis is important and will, in the future, permit the delivery of specific therapy. Broad-spectrum intravenous antibiotics should be avoided in patients with RSV bronchiolitis, as serious bacterial coinfections are uncommon [114]. In addition, accurate diagnosis helps in the institution of appropriate infection control measures and in facilitation of discharge planning [115]. RSV detection can be performed using culture and nonculture methods, the latter consisting of either antigen or nucleic acid detection.

Viral culture

The use of cell lines to propagate the virus is a long-established technique for diagnosis of RSV infection. Traditional tube culture is efficient and comprehensive, allowing strain typing and genetic characterisation, as well as antiviral susceptibility testing [116, 117]. The 3–7-day turnaround time, however, is more suitable for research studies or the investigation of complex cases and during outbreaks.

The clinical sample can also be centrifuged on to a single layer of cells using the shell vial culture method or by the use of a cluster tray of vials, which can reduce processing time to 1–2 days making it more useful for patient management [118]. Due to the labour-intensive nature and technical expertise required for the technique, it is mainly restricted to reference laboratories and large teaching hospitals [6, 7]. The labile nature of RSV also means that the virus can lose infectivity rapidly unless there is proper storage and rapid transport of specimens for laboratory testing.

Antigen detection

Antigen detection relies on identifying RSV antigenic fragments by viewing fluorescently labelled proteins under a microscope (direct immunofluorescence assay (DFA)) or using a commercially available rapid antigen detection test (RADT) [119]. A DFA has the advantage of ensuring a higher degree of accuracy in identifying the organism and can be performed in <1 h but requires expertise in reviewing specimens [117]. It has a reported sensitivity and specificity of up to 94% and 96%, respectively, when compared with real-time PCR [120].

RADTs include enzyme immunosorbent assays and chromatographic immunoassays, and have broad appeal due to their ease of use and applicability as a point-of-care test, with turnaround times of as little as 10 min, allowing early delivery of appropriate therapy [119]. However, a Cochrane review of RCTs, which included 759 children presenting to emergency departments with febrile illness and respiratory symptoms, concluded that, while the use of rapid viral testing reduced radiological investigations, it did not have any impact on the length of visit to the emergency department [121]. Overall, antigen detection tests have a range of 80–90% sensitivity in comparison with culture but are prone to higher false-positive rates outside of the peak RSV season and are considerably less reliable in older children and adults, who have reduced viral load compared with young children [122–124]. Thus, older children and adults may benefit from use of either culture or nucleic acid amplification testing to detect RSV.

Nucleic acid detection

Molecular tools, such as nucleic acid amplification testing, have transformed the ability to identify causative organisms in ARIs and have the distinct advantages of both speed and accuracy over viral culture and RADTs, respectively [4, 117]. Despite this, only 15% of laboratories in the USA use the technique, which costs US$35–125 for each sample tested (*versus* US$2–7 for DFA and US$4 for culture [116]), and have the equipment and specialist skills required [124].

RT-PCR has been proven to be as sensitive as culture in detecting RSV in hospital [125, 126] and community [5, 8] settings, in both adults and children. This technique has also been used to highlight minimal asymptomatic carriage of RSV in the community, making it a more useful method of accurately diagnosing the disease in this setting [127]. Further automation of such techniques will enable even more rapid, high-throughput handling of clinical specimens.

In the field of microbiology, molecular detection methods (rather than the slower culture-based methods, which often fail to detect a significant number of organisms) have revolutionised the detection of bacterial pathogens and have helped to identify distinct anatomical microbiomes. Similarly, the development of rapid multiplex PCR-based technology that can be deployed as a point-of-care test is likely to institute a paradigm shift in the diagnosis of viral pathogens at an earlier stage of illness. This can be of particular benefit in those at-risk groups (pre-term infants, the elderly and those with multiple comorbidities) who need early intervention or hospital admission [119]. A study of more than 430 clinical specimens validated the usefulness of this approach with the use of a 19-valent multiplex PCR test, which included RSV, and which demonstrated a mean sensitivity of 93% and specificity of 99% [128]. With the costs of multiplexing declining, this could also be a promising approach for community-based epidemiological studies [129]. Nonetheless, issues remain about the correlation between detection of the viral nucleic acids and clinical symptoms [130], and multiple respiratory virus detection from the same patient may be indicative of the presence of chronic lung disease rather than the severity of the infection [131].

A comparison of the available laboratory techniques for RSV diagnosis in terms of speed, expertise required and relative cost is shown in figure 4.

Anatomical sampling

Nasopharyngeal aspirates (NPAs) have traditionally been the gold standard in diagnosing RSV infection [132], but head-to-head comparisons of nasal swab sampling *versus* NPAs have shown equivalent results for most respiratory viruses [133, 134]. Swabs are prone to lower detection rates, which may be due to the lower volume of sample present on them.

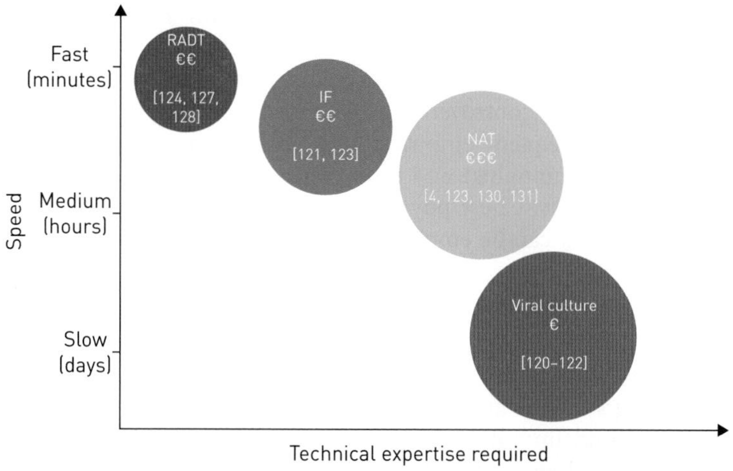

Figure 4. Comparison of laboratory techniques to diagnose RSV. The figure represents estimates and is not to scale. The size of the circles represents the relative sensitivity of each test in detecting RSV. Relative approximate costs are represented as € and are for reagents [116]. Numbers in square brackets indicate the relevant references. RADT: rapid antigen detection test; IF: immunofluorescence; NAT: nucleic acid testing (PCR).

Flocked nasal swabs have a better ability than NPAs to detect RSV, due to their effect of dislodging virus-infected epithelial cells from the mucosa [4]. They may be more suited to the outpatient setting, as they appear to be better tolerated than NPAs [135] and are also superior to nasal washes [136]. Swabs can be considered for routine testing in the community, but for hospitalised patients or if strain typing is required, an NPA is more appropriate.

In immunocompromised patients, nasal washes have very poor sensitivity in detecting RSV, probably due to lower viral load, with these patients benefiting from lower airway sampling [137]. The use of serology in diagnosing RSV in children is limited by the passive transfer of maternal antibodies, and is not useful in adults due to the persistence of antibodies from repeat infections.

Antiviral therapy and other potential treatments

Despite significant interest in disease-modifying therapies for RSV, the mainstay of treatment remains supportive. For the majority of affected children and adults, the illness is self-limiting, and simple measures, such as hydration and antipyretics, are sufficient. In those in whom symptoms are more severe, intensive supportive treatment in a supervised hospital environment may be required [96].

Supportive treatment

The most recent guidelines from the AAP [113] and the National Institute for Health and Care Excellence (NICE) [138] in the UK focus primarily on appropriate delivery of supplemental oxygen and hydration (table 1). Both guidelines advise delivery of supplemental oxygen using noninvasive and positive-pressure ventilation strategies, as well as *i.v.* or nasogastric fluids if oral hydration is insufficient. In addition, NICE recommends consideration of upper airway suctioning in children with respiratory distress, feeding difficulties or apnoea. Unlike the NICE guidance, the AAP recommends nebulised saline as an optional treatment in children with an expected length of hospital stay >72 h [113]. This strategy has generated some controversy, as the evidence base for its benefit has been conflicting. Despite their frequent empirical use, no recommendation is made regarding antipyretics (such as acetaminophen and ibuprofen), antitussives or decongestants by any of the most recent guidelines. Chest physiotherapy has not been recommended, although NICE adds the caveat that it can be employed if children have relevant comorbidities [138].

Antivirals and other pharmacotherapy

A variety of additional therapeutic agents have been used empirically for the treatment of bronchiolitis, including systemic and inhaled corticosteroids, nebulised bronchodilators and nebulised adrenaline. Guidelines now recommend that clinicians do not use these therapies in the treatment of children with bronchiolitis [96]. Antibiotic use is still permitted according to the AAP guidelines if there is evidence of bacterial coinfection, but this recommendation is not made elsewhere [139]. In adults with an RSV-associated exacerbation of underlying lung disease, the use of nebulised bronchodilators and oral corticosteroids remains commonplace. Some commentators argue that there is a theoretical risk that immunosuppression in this group of patients may potentiate the severity of viral infection *via* defects in humoral immunity [140], but the evidence is poor.

Ribavirin is currently the only licensed antiviral for the treatment of RSV in children, but the evidence is poor [141]. Consequently, most current guidelines make either no recommendation or do not recommend its routine use, which is also limited by its toxicity, including to healthcare workers [64, 141]. In adults, ribavirin is used off license and is usually reserved for those with severe immunocompromise such as haematopoietic stem cell transplant recipients [142], although the evidence base for its use is weak. In studies examining the effect of ribavirin (nebulised or systemic) in immunocompromised patients with RSV infection, there were trends towards improved outcomes, with reduced progression to lower respiratory tract involvement and less all-cause mortality [27]. However, none of these studies was sufficiently powered or robustly designed for definite conclusions to be drawn. The value of concomitant *i.v.* immunoglobulin administration alongside ribavirin also remains unproven [141].

Table 1. Current evidence for therapeutic options in managing RSV bronchiolitis

Supportive	**Inconclusive**	**Not supportive**
Oxygen	Ribavirin	Nebulised bronchodilators
Ventilation (invasive and noninvasive)	Nebulised hypertonic saline	Nebulised adrenaline
Nasogastric/*i.v.* fluids if unable to maintain oral intake	Upper airway suctioning	Steroids (oral/inhaled)
Palivizumab for prevention in high-risk babies	Azithromycin	Antibiotics without evidence of bacterial infection
	IVIG	Montelukast

Based on guidelines published by the American Academy of Pediatrics [113], The National Institute of Health and Care Excellence [138] and reference [96]. IVIG: *i.v.* immunoglobulin.

Immunoglobulins, both RSV-specific and nonspecific, have also been used in the treatment of RSV-related bronchiolitis in children. Like many other therapeutic interventions, the evidence base for this remains weak, and a Cochrane review in 2006 concluded that there was no statistically significant benefit of such treatment [143].

Montelukast, a leukotriene inhibitor used in the treatment of asthma, has also been tried in the treatment of bronchiolitis. A 2015 Cochrane review considered five randomised control trials comparing montelukast treatment with placebo in children <2 years of age with a diagnosis of bronchiolitis. Two of the five studies examined the impact of montelukast acutely during the hospital admission, whereas the other three studies focused on longer-term use over several weeks following a diagnosis of bronchiolitis to prevent ongoing episodes of wheeze. The authors concluded that, while none of the studies demonstrated a difference between montelukast and placebo, no definite conclusions could be drawn due to statistical inconsistencies and the weaknesses of the studies [144].

Azithromycin, a macrolide antibiotic with immunomodulatory properties, was shown to have no impact on clinical outcome measures, such as duration of hospital stay, oxygen supplementation or symptom scores, when given to infants during acute RSV bronchiolitis [64]. It was, however, found to reduce levels of neutrophilic inflammation in the airways of mice in a murine bronchiolitis model [145]. A proof-of-concept study was therefore conducted in human infants investigating the effectiveness of azithromycin compared with placebo at reducing post-bronchiolitis wheeze and chronic airway inflammation in previously healthy infants aged 1–18 months [146]. The results demonstrated that treatment with azithromycin for 14 days during the acute bronchiolitic illness prolonged the time to a third parent-reported wheezing episode and reduced the overall number of days with respiratory symptoms in the 50 weeks post-treatment [146]. However, the primary clinical outcome of a reduction in the number of children experiencing two or more wheezing episodes was not met, and the proportion of participants diagnosed with asthma during the follow-up period was also no different [146]. More promising were the findings of a 2007 double-blind placebo-controlled study from Turkey investigating the use of clarithromycin in infants (<7 months of age) hospitalised with RSV bronchiolitis. Statistically significant reductions in length of stay, the need for supplemental oxygen and bronchodilation were reported, in addition to fewer re-admissions with wheeze in the subsequent 6 months. However, this study had a small sample size, and further studies would be needed to validate the findings [147].

Several new therapeutic agents are currently in the development pipeline. These fall broadly into four different groups: small interfering RNA, immunoglobulins, fusion inhibitors and small molecules [96]. Each aims to disrupt the production or action of proteins produced by RSV, and thus limit its pathogenicity. Agents that have demonstrated efficacy include ALN-RSV01, which uses antisense mechanisms to disrupt viral protein synthesis and thus viral replication. Proof-of-concept studies in healthy adults inoculated experimentally with RSV demonstrated reduced infection rates with concomitant use of intranasal ALN-RSV01 [148], and use of the compound in lung transplant patients with RSV infection has been shown to reduce the rate of new or progressive bronchiolitis obliterans syndrome at 180 days post-infection [149].

Promising results have also been seen with the fusion inhibitor GS-5806, which reduced the viral load and severity of clinical disease in a double-blind placebo-controlled viral challenge study in healthy adult volunteers [150]. More recently, a placebo-controlled trial of a second antiviral (ALS-008176, which acts on the RSV polymerase L protein and inhibits viral replication in infected cells) enhanced viral clearance and reduced disease severity. Importantly, this compound appeared to be effective even when administration was delayed until 12 h after virus detection [151].

Vaccines and prevention of RSV

The lack of effective, disease-specific therapies for RSV, alongside the significant global burden and cost of the disease, has stimulated huge interest and research in vaccine discovery. However, the development of RSV vaccines has been hampered by a number of factors. First, defects in both innate and adaptive neonatal immune responses make infantile vaccination problematic. In addition, the presence of maternal antibodies, despite offering valuable protection to the newborn child, may suppress the development of intrinsic antibody responses [152].

Although certain immunisation strategies are effective in neonates (*e.g.* bacilli Calmette–Guérin for tuberculosis), many vaccines require repeated boosters and/or are delayed until the child's immune system is more mature [153]. In addition to the challenges posed by the host response, RSV as a pathogen creates difficulties for vaccine development. In particular, natural infection does not result in durable immunity, even in adults, and re-infection with an identical strain of virus is commonplace [85]. A successful vaccine therefore needs to induce immune responses more potently than the natural infection, while simultaneously preventing an excessive and pathological inflammatory response in the host.

Unfortunately, this balance was not achieved by early vaccine attempts. In the 1960s, a formalin-inactivated vaccine was developed for use in infants and children. Although a similar approach was effective and safe with poliovirus immunisation, it resulted in an insufficient neutralising antibody response and enhanced disease during subsequent natural infection. In one trial, nearly 80% of naturally infected vaccinated children required hospitalisation, and two died [154]. As a result, progress in RSV vaccination development has been intensely cautious and slow.

Strategies to enable the investigation of the immune response both to natural infection with RSV and to a variety of potential vaccines have frequently relied on the use of animal models. Unfortunately, no single model has been sufficient to replicate the situation in human infection [155]. The use of human RSV challenge has considerable advantages over animal models, but this too remains imperfect. Adults are not the primary target of RSV vaccines designed to prevent infantile bronchiolitis, although there may be a role for vaccination of pregnant women, adult care-givers and those adults at risk of severe RSV disease. However, challenge studies are currently limited to normal healthy adults, and infants, pregnant women, the immunocompromised and frail adults cannot be subjected to experimental infection. Ultimately, a single vaccination strategy for all target groups is unlikely to be preferred [155].

Despite these hurdles, a large number of potential vaccines are under development, and the likelihood of one or more successful vaccine(s) reaching the market within the next decade is high [6, 155]. These vaccines fall into four broad categories: live attenuated, subunit, vector based and particulate. Each targets different mechanisms of immunogenicity and thus would potentially suit different groups of at-risk individuals. Strategies for optimising the effect of vaccines include the use of maternal vaccination to enable passive transfer of immunity *via* immunoglobulins to levels sufficient to provide effective protection in an otherwise poorly immunogenic infant. Immunisation would need to be delivered to the mother in the second or third trimester for the transfer of passive immunisation to be optimal [152], which would be of less value for premature infants in whom *trans*-placental antibody transfer is inefficient. Immunisation of individuals in contact with vulnerable groups, such as healthcare or nursery workers, or older siblings, may be another viable alternative to reduce virus transmission rates through herd immunity.

Live attenuated vaccines show promise in infants, as they may safely induce local protective immunity. They may, however, be of limited immunogenicity, and the possibility of pathological responses in (undiagnosed) immunodeficient states remains a concern [153]. Nevertheless, some success has been achieved, and a variety of phase 1 and 2 clinical trials are currently underway. The leading contender in the field is MEDI-559 (MedImmune/National Institute of Allergy and Infectious Diseases, Bethesda, MD, USA). This vaccine has been well tolerated by healthy children and infants, with the majority of participants mounting a detectable serological response or shedding the vaccine virus, as detected by PCR [7]. Trials of other live-attenuated vaccines are ongoing (clinicaltrials.gov identifier numbers: NCT02040831, NCT01893554 and NCT01852266). Advantages of live attenuated vaccines include their ability to be delivered intranasally, to replicate even in the presence of passively delivered maternal antibody and to stimulate multiple components of the immune system [152]. Despite these attributes, the potential for reversion to wild type and for secondary transmission from a vaccinated child to contacts, as well as the difficulty in producing sufficient attenuation, has slowed progression towards clinical use [155].

Some of these issues could be avoided with the use of subunit vaccines, which have no potential for infectivity in either vaccinees or their contacts. Unfortunately, they often fail to stimulate a sufficient response in the immature infant immune system [96], and their optimal use may prove to be in boosting the adult response. Subunit vaccines, which contain purified proteins with or without the addition of immune-stimulating adjuvants, have been shown to be effective in inducing neutralising antibodies in the serum of adults [156] and may offer an effective option for the elderly and pregnant women [96]. In seronegative individuals, there is a possible risk of vaccine-enhanced disease, and hence these vaccines are unlikely to be useful in previously unexposed neonates. Particle-based vaccines, which consist of multiple proteins arranged on virus/bacteria-like structures, mimic infective agents and may be able to induce durable immunity [155]. Vector-based

Table 2. Outstanding questions in the field

What innate and adaptive immune mechanisms determine the susceptibility of infants to bronchiolitis?
Why do some people with RSV develop symptoms, while others remain asymptomatic?
Why is it possible for adults (and children) to be re-infected with the same strain of RSV?
What explains the variable findings with respect to the association between RSV and wheeze in later life?
What are the best correlates of protection to use in vaccine studies?
What are the ideal qualities of vaccines that target specific risk groups (*i.e.* pregnant women, adult care-givers, school-aged children and elderly persons)?
How can animal models be improved further?
What public health measures are appropriate and feasible in resource-limited settings?

vaccines use other viruses or bacteria as a means of delivery of RSV genetic components. Viral protein production allows antigens to be made within the host, while the vector is rendered harmless [155].

Much of the recent progress in vaccine development is due to improvements in our understanding of the structure and function of RSV, the immunogens that it makes, and the protective and harmful immune responses that these raise in the host. A detailed appreciation of the host immune response to RSV, particularly the T- and B-cell immune responses, is vital to future vaccine development.

Strategies for prevention of RSV focus mainly on the use of passive immunisation. Palivizumab, a humanised mAb against RSV, is licensed for use in high-risk babies during RSV season to prevent disease in the lower respiratory tract. Large RCTs in the late 1990s showed a reduction of 55% in the rate of hospitalisation for RSV in pre-term infants treated

Table 3. Key take-home messages

- RSV is the leading cause of bronchiolitis in infants and excess winter deaths in the elderly.
- RSV is estimated to cause 30 million ARIs in children and in excess of 60 000 deaths worldwide each year.
- RSV causes upper and lower respiratory tract infections in both children and adults. Infants and young children, the frail elderly and those with chronic cardiorespiratory disease or immunocompromise are at greatest risk of morbidity and mortality.
- RSV disease is predominantly a winter illness. Infection incidence peaks in December to January in northern European countries and in February to March in southern Europe.
- Susceptibility to severe RSV disease is increased by exposure to tobacco smoke, air pollution, crowding (in day-care, nursing homes or hospitals) and the presence of school-aged older siblings.
- RSV infection in children has been linked to the development of asthma and atopy, although a causal relationship remains unproven.
- RSV has been classified into two distinct subgroups (A and B) based on antigenic variability, with the suggestion that subtype A causes more severe disease. Genetic sequence analysis is the most accurate way of identifying viral subtypes for research purposes.
- A key characteristic of RSV is its ability to evade immunity and thus to re-infect, despite limited antigenic variation.
- Laboratory diagnosis of RSV is not essential but can facilitate appropriate antibiotic stewardship.
- A nasopharyngeal aspirate is the gold standard for collection of samples, with flocked nasal swabs an acceptable alternative in community settings. Immunocompromised patients should have lower airway sampling and PCR diagnosis to increase the chances of a positive result.
- Culture remains the gold standard for diagnosing RSV but is being overtaken by fast molecular techniques. Rapid antigen detection kits are relatively inexpensive and are easy for point-of-care testing, but limited by lower sensitivity and poor reliability in adults. Nucleic acid detection (PCR) now offers high sensitivity and increasingly quick turnaround times.
- Hand decontamination with alcohol or soap is important in preventing nosocomial transmission.
- Appropriate supportive treatment with fluids, oxygenation and ventilatory support remains the cornerstone of RSV management.
- Salbutamol, adrenaline and systemic corticosteroids should not be routinely administered to infants with bronchiolitis.
- There are several very promising antiviral drugs and vaccines in development, but their impact in clinical settings is currently difficult to anticipate. Promising vaccination strategies include the use of maternal vaccines, inactivated or live vaccines for neonates and subunit vaccines for the elderly.

with palivizumab compared with placebo [157]. Further studies have confirmed its efficacy, and the AAP has recently produced advice as to which at-risk infants benefit from treatment [158]. Monthly administration of antibody is costly, which largely limits its use, and it is of no value in established infection [155].

As discussed above, the potential benefits of RSV prevention with passive antibody could extend beyond the effect on acute morbidity and mortality, with possible impacts on the occurrence of longer-term sequelae, such as recurrent wheeze [97]. Of the newer mAb candidates, motavizumab seemed the most promising [99]; however, its development has been halted due to nonsuperiority to palivizumab and adverse skin reactions. It is to be hoped that other mAbs can be marketed for RSV prevention at lower cost.

Conclusion

A summary of some of the outstanding questions in the field of RSV research are outlined in table 2 and the key take-home messages of the current research on RSV are outlined in table 3. RSV infection is currently ubiquitous during early childhood, causing a vast burden of disease throughout the world. The link between severe childhood infections and the development of longer-term respiratory ill health is intriguing but as yet poorly mapped and understood, and the proposed causal link between bronchiolitis, the later development of recurrent infantile wheeze and the diagnosis of childhood asthma remains to be established with certainty. While infections with many common and important respiratory pathogens (*e.g.* influenza virus, *H. influenza* and *Streptococcus pneumoniae*) are preventable with vaccines, RSV has so far eluded vaccinologists. There is now a race among those developing a large number of vaccines that aim to induce long-lasting protection. Field trials of both vaccines and antiviral drugs in real-life settings are keenly awaited, but for now the treatment of RSV disease remains largely supportive. The advent of antivirals and vaccines that reduce viral load and disease, coupled with increasingly sensitive molecular techniques to diagnose infection at an early stage, will potentially greatly reduce the global impact of RSV infection in the near future. Ultimately, such measures may have an impact on the ability of RSV to circulate in communities, changing the population dynamics of infection and altering the global grip of this virus.

References

1. Nair H, Nokes DJ, Gessner BD, *et al.* Global burden of acute lower respiratory infections due to respiratory syncytial virus in young children: a systematic review and meta-analysis. *Lancet* 2010; 375: 1545–1555.
2. Sigurs N, Aljassim F, Kjellman B, *et al.* Asthma and allergy patterns over 18 years after severe RSV bronchiolitis in the first year of life. *Thorax* 2010; 65: 1045–1052.
3. Carbonell-Estrany X, Pérez-Yarza EG, García LS, *et al.* Long-term burden and respiratory effects of respiratory syncytial virus hospitalization in preterm infants – the SPRING Study. *PloS One* 2015; 10: e0125422.
4. Popow-Kraupp T, Aberle JH. Diagnosis of respiratory syncytial virus infection. *Open Microbiol J* 2011; 5: 128–134.
5. Falsey AR, Formica MA, Walsh EE. Diagnosis of respiratory syncytial virus infection: comparison of reverse transcription-PCR to viral culture and serology in adults with respiratory illness. *J Clin Microbiol* 2002; 40: 817–820.
6. Jaberolansar N, Toth I, Young PR, *et al.* Recent advances in the development of subunit-based RSV vaccines. *Expert Rev Vaccines* 2016; 15: 53–68.
7. Malkin E, Yogev R, Abughali N, *et al.* Safety and immunogenicity of a live attenuated RSV vaccine in healthy RSV-seronegative children 5 to 24 months of age. *PloS One* 2013; 8: e77104.
8. Hall CB, Weinberg GA, Iwane MK, *et al.* The burden of respiratory syncytial virus infection in young children. *N Engl J Med* 2009; 360: 588–598.

9. Branche AR, Falsey AR. Respiratory syncytial virus infection in older adults: an under-recognized problem. *Drugs Aging* 2015; 32: 261–269.
10. Falsey AR, Hennessey PA, Formica MA, *et al.* Respiratory syncytial virus infection in elderly and high-risk adults. *N Engl J Med* 2005; 352: 1749–1759.
11. Thompson WW, Shay DK, Weintraub E, *et al.* Mortality associated with influenza and respiratory syncytial virus in the United States. *JAMA* 2003; 289: 179–186.
12. Zambon MC, Stockton JD, Clewley JP, *et al.* Contribution of influenza and respiratory syncytial virus to community cases of influenza-like illness: an observational study. *Lancet* 2001; 358: 1410–1416.
13. Tang JW, Loh TP. Correlations between climate factors and incidence – a contributor to RSV seasonality. *Rev Med Virol* 2014; 24: 15–34.
14. Tran DN, Trinh QD, Pham NTK, *et al.* Clinical and epidemiological characteristics of acute respiratory virus infections in Vietnamese children. *Epidemiol Infect* 2015; 144: 1–10.
15. Bloom-Feshbach K, Alonso WJ, Charu V, *et al.* Latitudinal variations in seasonal activity of influenza and respiratory syncytial virus (RSV): a global comparative review. *PLoS One* 2013; 8: e54445.
16. Simoes EAF. Environmental and demographic risk factors for respiratory syncytial virus lower respiratory tract disease. *J Pediatr* 2003; 143: Suppl., S118–S126.
17. Constantopoulos A, Kafetzis D, Syrogiannopoulos G, *et al.* Burden of respiratory syncytial viral infections on paediatric hospitals: a two-year prospective epidemiological study. *Eur J Clin Microbiol Infect Dis* 2002; 21: 102–107.
18. Shaw Stewart PD. Seasonality and selective trends in viral acute respiratory tract infections. *Med Hypotheses* 2015; 86: 104–119.
19. Rudan I, Boschi-Pinto C, Biloglav Z, *et al.* Epidemiology and etiology of childhood pneumonia. *Bull World Health Organ* 2008; 86: 408–416.
20. Simoes EA. Respiratory syncytial virus infection. *Lancet* 1999; 354: 847–852.
21. Moyes J, Cohen C, Pretorius M, *et al.* Epidemiology of respiratory syncytial virus-associated acute lower respiratory tract infection hospitalizations among HIV-infected and HIV-uninfected South African children, 2010–2011. *J Infect Dis* 2013; 208: Suppl. 3, S217–S226.
22. Collins PL, Graham BS. Viral and host factors in human respiratory syncytial virus pathogenesis. *J Virol* 2008; 82: 2040–2055.
23. Sommer C, Resch B, Simões EAF. Risk factors for severe respiratory syncytial virus lower respiratory tract infection. *Open Microbiol J* 2011; 5: 144–154.
24. Fleming DM, Taylor RJ, Lustig RL, *et al.* Modelling estimates of the burden of respiratory syncytial virus infection in adults and the elderly in the United Kingdom. *BMC Infect Dis* 2015; 15: 443.
25. Falsey AR, McElhaney JE, Beran J, *et al.* Respiratory syncytial virus and other respiratory viral infections in older adults with moderate to severe influenza-like illness. *J Infect Dis* 2014; 209: 1873–1881.
26. Madhi SA, Venter M, Madhi A, *et al.* Differing manifestations of respiratory syncytial virus-associated severe lower respiratory tract infections in human immunodeficiency virus type 1-infected and uninfected children. *Pediatr Infect Dis J* 2001; 20: 164–170.
27. Shah JN, Chemaly RF. Management of RSV infections in adult recipients of hematopoietic stem cell transplantation. *Blood* 2011; 117: 2755–2763.
28. Shah DP, Ghantoji SS, Mulanovich VE, *et al.* Management of respiratory viral infections in hematopoietic cell transplant recipients. *Am J Blood Res* 2012; 2: 203–218.
29. Blount RE, Morris JA, Savage RE. Recovery of cytopathogenic agent from chimpanzees with coryza. *Proc Soc Exper Biol Med* 1956; 92: 544–549.
30. Chanock R, Finberg L. Recovery from infants with respiratory illness of a virus related to chimpanzee coryza agent (CCA). II. Epidemiologic aspects of infection in infants and young children. *Am J Hyg* 1957; 66: 291–300.
31. Mufson MA, Orvell C, Rafnar B, *et al.* Two distinct subtypes of human respiratory syncytial virus. *J Gen Virol* 1985; 66: 2111–2124.
32. Johnson SM, McNally BA, Ioannidis I, *et al.* Respiratory syncytial virus uses CX3CR1 as a receptor on primary human airway epithelial cultures. *Plos Pathogen* 2015; 11: e1005318.
33. Levine S, Kaliaber-Franco R, Paradiso PR. Demonstration that glycoprotein G is the attachment protein of respiratory syncytial virus. *J Gen Virol* 1987; 68: 2521–2524.
34. Sullender WM. Respiratory syncytial virus genetic and antigenic diversity. *Clin Microbiol Rev* 2000; 13: 1–15.
35. Tan L, Lemey P, Houspie L, *et al.* Genetic variability among complete human respiratory syncytial virus subgroup A genomes: bridging molecular evolutionary dynamics and epidemiology. *PLoS One* 2012; 7: e51439.
36. Bächi T, Howe C. Morphogenesis and ultrastructure of respiratory syncytial virus. *J Virol* 1973; 12: 1173–1180.
37. Gan SW, Tan E, Lin X, *et al.* The small hydrophobic protein of the human respiratory syncytial virus forms pentameric ion channels. *J Biol Chem* 2012; 287: 24671–24689.
38. Gower TL, Pastey MK, Peeples ME, *et al.* RhoA signaling is required for respiratory syncytial virus-induced syncytium formation and filamentous virion morphology. *J Virol* 2005; 79: 5326–5336.

39. Kwilas S, Liesman RM, Zhang L, *et al.* Respiratory syncytial virus grown in Vero cells contains a truncated attachment protein that alters its infectivity and dependence on glycosaminoglycans. *J Virol* 2009; 83: 10710–10718.
40. Gould PS, Easton AJ. Coupled translation of the second open reading frame of M2 mRNA is sequence dependent and differs significantly within the subfamily Pneumovirinae. *J Virol* 2007; 81: 8488–8496.
41. Mitra R, Baviskar P, Duncan-Decocq RR, *et al.* The human respiratory syncytial virus matrix protein is required for maturation of viral filaments. *J Virol* 2012; 86: 4432–4443.
42. Thorburn K, Kerr S, Taylor N, *et al.* RSV outbreak in a paediatric intensive care unit. *J Hosp Infect* 2004; 57: 194–201.
43. Bont L. Nosocomial RSV infection control and outbreak management. *Paediatr Respir Rev* 2009; 10: Suppl. 1, 16–17.
44. Hall CB. Respiratory syncytial virus and parainfluenza virus. *N Engl J Med* 2001; 344: 1917–1928.
45. Jensen C, Johnson FB. Comparison of various transport media for viability maintenance of herpes simplex virus, respiratory syncytial virus, and adenovirus. *Diagn Microbiol Infect Dis* 1994; 19: 137–142.
46. Persson BD, Jaffe AB, Fearns R, *et al.* Respiratory syncytial virus can infect basal cells and alter human airway epithelial differentiation. *Plos One* 2014; 9: e102368.
47. Wu W, Munday DC, Howell G, *et al.* Characterization of the interaction between human respiratory syncytial virus and the cell cycle in continuous cell culture and primary human airway epithelial cells. *J Virol* 2011; 85: 10300–10309.
48. Collins PL, Graham BS. Viral and host factors in human respiratory syncytial virus pathogenesis. *J Virol* 2008; 82: 2040–2055.
49. DiFranza JR, Masaquel A, Barrett AM, *et al.* Systematic literature review assessing tobacco smoke exposure as a risk factor for serious respiratory syncytial virus disease among infants and young children. *BMC Pediatr* 2012; 12: 81.
50. Harrod KS, Jaramillo RJ, Rosenberger CL, *et al.* Increased susceptibility to RSV infection by exposure to inhaled diesel engine emissions. *Am J Respir Cell Mol Biol* 2003; 28: 451–463.
51. DeVincenzo JP, Wilkinson T, Vaishnaw A, *et al.* Viral load drives disease in humans experimentally infected with respiratory syncytial virus. *Am J Respir Crit Care Med* 2010; 182: 1305–1314.
52. El Saleeby CM, Bush AJ, Harrison LM, *et al.* Respiratory syncytial virus load, viral dynamics, and disease severity in previously healthy naturally infected children. *J Infect Dis* 2011; 204: 996–1002.
53. Bukreyev A, Yang L, Fricke J, *et al.* The secreted form of respiratory syncytial virus G glycoprotein helps the virus evade antibody-mediated restriction of replication by acting as an antigen decoy and through effects on Fc receptor-bearing leukocytes. *J Virol* 2008; 82: 12191–12204.
54. Tripp RA, Jones LP, Haynes LM, *et al.* CX3C chemokine mimicry by respiratory syncytial virus G glycoprotein. *Nat Immunol* 2001; 2: 732–738.
55. Van Drunen Littel-Van Den Hurk S, Watkiss ER. Pathogenesis of respiratory syncytial virus. *Curr Opin Virol* 2012; 2: 300–305.
56. Collins PL, Melero JA. Progress in understanding and controlling respiratory syncytial virus: still crazy after all these years. *Virus Res* 2011; 162: 80–99.
57. Thomsen SF, Stensballe LG, Skytthe A, *et al.* Increased concordance of severe respiratory syncytial virus infection in identical twins. *Pediatrics* 2008; 121: 493–496.
58. Miyairi I, DeVincenzo JP. Human genetic factors and respiratory syncytial virus disease severity. *Clin Microbiol Rev* 2008; 21: 686–703.
59. Yoo J-K, Kim TS, Hufford MM, *et al.* Viral infection of the lung: host response and sequelae. *J Allergy Clin Immunol* 2013; 132: 1263–1276.
60. Peebles RS, Graham BS. Pathogenesis of respiratory syncytial virus infection in the murine model. *Proc Am Thorac Soc* 2005; 2: 110–115.
61. Goritzka M, Makris S, Kausar F, *et al.* Alveolar macrophage-derived type I interferons orchestrate innate immunity to RSV through recruitment of antiviral monocytes. *J Exp Med* 2015; 212: 699–714.
62. Rossi GA, Colin AA. Infantile respiratory syncytial virus and human rhinovirus infections: respective role in inception and persistence of wheezing. *Eur Respir J* 2015; 45: 774–789.
63. Openshaw PJ, Tregoning JS. Immune responses and disease enhancement during respiratory syncytial virus infection. *Clin Microbiol Rev* 2005; 18: 541–555.
64. Tregoning JS, Schwarze J. Respiratory viral infections in infants: causes, clinical symptoms, virology, and immunology. *Clin Microbiol Rev* 2010; 23: 74–98.
65. Eisenhut M. Extrapulmonary manifestations of severe respiratory syncytial virus infection – a systematic review. *Crit Care* 2006; 10: R107.
66. Culley FJ, Pennycook AMJ, Tregoning JS, *et al.* Differential chemokine expression following respiratory virus infection reflects Th1- or Th2-biased immunopathology. *J Virol* 2006; 80: 4521–4527.
67. Legg JP, Hussain IR, Warner JA, *et al.* Type 1 and type 2 cytokine imbalance in acute respiratory syncytial virus bronchiolitis. *Am J Respir Crit Care Med* 2003; 168: 633–639.
68. Sumino K, Tucker J, Shahab M, *et al.* Antiviral IFN-γ responses of monocytes at birth predict respiratory tract illness in the first year of life. *J Allergy Clin Immunol* 2012; 129: 1267–1273.
69. Tal G, Mandelberg A, Dalal I, *et al.* Association between common Toll-like receptor 4 mutations and severe respiratory syncytial virus disease. *J Infect Dis* 2004; 189: 2057–2063.

70. Hoebee B, Rietveld E, Bont L, *et al.* Association of severe respiratory syncytial virus bronchiolitis with interleukin-4 and interleukin-4 receptor alpha polymorphisms. *J Infect Dis* 2003; 187: 2–11.
71. Hull J, Thomson A, Kwiatkowski D. Association of respiratory syncytial virus bronchiolitis with the interleukin 8 gene region in UK families. *Thorax* 2000; 55: 1023–1027.
72. Kollmann TR, Levy O, Montgomery RR, *et al.* Innate immune function by Toll-like receptors: distinct responses in newborns and the elderly. *Immunity* 2012; 37: 771–783.
73. Abraha HY, Lanctôt KL, Paes B. Risk of respiratory syncytial virus infection in preterm infants: reviewing the need for prevention. *Expert Rev Respir Med* 2015; 9: 779–799.
74. Chu HY, Steinhoff MC, Magaret A, *et al.* Respiratory syncytial virus transplacental antibody transfer and kinetics in mother–infant pairs in Bangladesh. *J Infect Dis* 2014; 210: 1582–1589.
75. Hall CB, Powell KR, MacDonald NE, *et al.* Respiratory syncytial viral infection in children with compromised immune function. *N Engl J Med* 1986; 315: 77–81.
76. Chandwani S, Borkowsky W, Krasinski K, *et al.* Respiratory syncytial virus infection in human immunodeficiency virus-infected children. *J Pediatr* 1990; 117: 251–254.
77. Openshaw PJM. Antiviral immune responses and lung inflammation after respiratory syncytial virus infection. *Proc Am Thorac Soc* 2005; 2: 121–125.
78. Loebbermann J, Schnoeller C, Thornton H, *et al.* IL-10 regulates viral lung immunopathology during acute respiratory syncytial virus infection in mice. *PLoS One* 2012; 7: e32371.
79. Cannon MJ, Openshaw PJ, Askonas BA. Cytotoxic T cells clear virus but augment lung pathology in mice infected with respiratory syncytial virus. *J Exp Med* 1988; 168: 1163–1168.
80. Spikiatkhachorn A, Braciale TJ. Virus-specific memory and effector T lymphocytes exhibit different cytokine responses to antigens during murine respiratory syncytial virus infection. *J Virol* 1997; 71: 678–685.
81. Jozwik A, Habibi MS, Paras A, *et al.* RSV-specific airway resident memory $CD8^+$ T cells and differential disease severity after experimental human infection. *Nature Commun* 2015; 6: 10224.
82. Shirey KA, Pletneva LM, Puche AC, *et al.* Control of RSV-induced lung injury by alternatively activated macrophages is IL-4Rα-, TLR4-, and IFN-β-dependent. *Mucosal Immunol* 2010; 3: 291–300.
83. Smit JJ, Rudd BD, Lukacs NW. Plasmacytoid dendritic cells inhibit pulmonary immunopathology and promote clearance of respiratory syncytial virus. *J Exp Med* 2006; 203: 1153–1159.
84. Habibi MS, Jozwik A, Makris S, *et al.* Impaired antibody-mediated protection and defective IgA B-cell memory in experimental infection of adults with respiratory syncytial virus. *Am J Respir Crit Care Med* 2015; 191: 1040–1049.
85. Hall CB, Walsh EE, Long CE, *et al.* Immunity to and frequency of reinfection with respiratory syncytial virus. *J Infect Dis* 1991; 163: 693–698.
86. Aberle JH, Aberle SW, Pracher E, *et al.* Single *versus* dual respiratory virus infections in hospitalized infants: impact on clinical course of disease and interferon-γ response. *Pediatr Infect Dis J* 2005; 24: 605–610.
87. Looney RJ, Falsey AR, Walsh E, *et al.* Effect of aging on cytokine production in response to respiratory syncytial virus infection. *J Infect Dis* 2002; 185: 682–685.
88. Cherukuri A, Patton K, Gasser RA, *et al.* Adults 65 years and older have reduced numbers of functional memory T cells to respiratory syncytial virus fusion (F) protein. *Clin Vaccine Immunol* 2012; 20: 239–247.
89. Openshaw PJ, Chiu C. Protective and dysregulated T cell immunity in RSV infection. *Curr Opin Virol* 2013; 3: 468–474.
90. Smyth RL, Openshaw PJM. Bronchiolitis. *Lancet* 2006; 368: 312–322.
91. Borchers AT, Chang C, Gershwin ME, *et al.* Respiratory syncytial virus – a comprehensive review. *Clin Rev Allergy Immunol* 2013; 45: 331–379.
92. Schroeder AR, Mansbach JM, Stevenson M, *et al.* Apnea in children hospitalized with bronchiolitis. *Pediatrics* 2013; 132: e1194–e1201.
93. Wright M, Piedimonte G. Respiratory syncytial virus prevention and therapy: past, present, and future. *Pediatr Pulmonol* 2011; 46: 324–347.
94. Meissner HC, Ingelfinger JR, Meissner HC. Viral bronchiolitis in children. *N Engl J Med* 2016; 374: 62–72.
95. Stein RT, Sherrill D, Morgan WJ, *et al.* Respiratory syncytial virus in early life and risk of wheeze and allergy by age 13 years. *Lancet* 1999; 354: 541–545.
96. Mazur NI, Martinón-Torres F, Baraldi E, *et al.* Lower respiratory tract infection caused by respiratory syncytial virus: current management and new therapeutics. *Lancet Respir Med* 2015; 3: 1–13.
97. Blanken MO, Rovers MM, Molenaar JM, *et al.* Respiratory syncytial virus and recurrent wheeze in healthy preterm infants. *N Engl J Med* 2013; 368: 1791–1799.
98. Carbonell-Estrany X, Simões EAF, Dagan R, *et al.* Motavizumab for prophylaxis of respiratory syncytial virus in high-risk children: a noninferiority trial. *Pediatrics* 2010; 125: e35–e51.
99. O'Brien KL, Chandran A, Weatherholtz R, *et al.* Efficacy of motavizumab for the prevention of respiratory syncytial virus disease in healthy Native American infants: a phase 3 randomised double-blind placebo-controlled trial. *Lancet Infect Dis* 2015; 15: 1398–1408.
100. Falsey AR, Walsh EE. Respiratory syncytial virus infection in adults. *Clin Microbiol Rev* 2000; 13: 371–384.

101. Sundaram ME, Meece JK, Sifakis F, *et al.* Medically attended respiratory syncytial virus infections in adults aged ⩾50 years: clinical characteristics and outcomes. *Clin Infect Dis* 2014; 58: 342–349.
102. Wald TG, Miller BA, Shult P, *et al.* Can respiratory syncytial virus and influenza A be distinguished clinically in institutionalized older persons? *J Am Geriatr Soc* 1995; 43: 170–174.
103. Hertz MI, Englund JA, Snover D, *et al.* Respiratory syncytial virus-induced acute lung injury in adult patients with bone marrow transplants: a clinical approach and review of the literature. *Medicine* 1989; 68: 269–281.
104. Harrington RD, Hooton TM, Hackman RC, *et al.* An outbreak of respiratory syncytial virus in a bone marrow transplant center. *J Infect Dis* 1992; 165: 987–993.
105. Falsey AR, Formica MA, Hennessey PA, *et al.* Detection of respiratory syncytial virus in adults with chronic obstructive pulmonary disease. *Am J Respir Crit Care Med* 2006; 173: 639–643.
106. Johnston SL, Pattemore PK, Sanderson G, *et al.* Community study of role of viral infections in exacerbations of asthma in 9-11 year old children. *BMJ* 1995; 310: 1225–1229.
107. Teichtahl H, Buckmaster N, Pertnikovs E. The incidence of respiratory tract infection in adults requiring hospitalization for asthma. *Chest* 1997; 112: 591–596.
108. Pelaez A, Lyon GM, Force SD, *et al.* Efficacy of oral ribavirin in lung transplant patients with respiratory syncytial virus lower respiratory tract infection. *J Heart Lung Transplant* 2009; 28: 67–71.
109. Hurst JR, Vestbo J, Anzueto A, *et al.* Susceptibility to exacerbation in chronic obstructive pulmonary disease. *N Engl J Med* 2010; 363: 1128–1138.
110. Shah PD, McDyer JF. Viral infections in lung transplant recipients. *Semin Respir Crit Care Med* 2010; 31: 243–254.
111. Schwarze J, O'Donnell DR, Rohwedder A, *et al.* Latency and persistence of respiratory syncytial virus despite T cell immunity. *Am J Respir Crit Care Med* 2004; 169: 801–805.
112. Falsey AR, Hennessey PA, Formica MA, *et al.* Respiratory syncytial virus infection in elderly and high-risk adults. *N Engl J Med* 2005; 352: 1749–1759.
113. Ralston S, Lieberthal A, Meissner H, *et al.* Clinical practice guideline: the diagnosis, management, and prevention of bronchiolitis. *Pediatrics* 2014; 134: e1474–e1502.
114. Purcell K, Fergie J. Concurrent serious bacterial infections in 912 infants and children hospitalized for treatment of respiratory syncytial virus lower respiratory tract infection. *Pediatr Infect Dis J* 2004; 23: 267–269.
115. Hall CB. Nosocomial respiratory syncytial virus infections: the 'Cold War' has not ended. *Clin Infect Dis* 2000; 31: 590–596.
116. Leland DS, Ginocchio CC. Role of cell culture for virus detection in the age of technology. *Clin Microbiol Rev* 2007; 20: 49–78.
117. Ginocchio CC, McAdam AJ. Current best practices for respiratory virus testing. *J Clin Microbiol* 2011; 49: Suppl., 44–48.
118. Matthey S, Nicholson D, Ruhs S, *et al.* Rapid detection of respiratory viruses by shell vial culture and direct staining by using pooled and individual monoclonal antibodies. *J Clin Microbiol* 1992; 30: 540–544.
119. Prendergast C, Papenburg J. Rapid antigen-based testing for respiratory syncytial virus: moving diagnostics from bench to bedside? *Future Microbiol* 2013; 8: 435–444.
120. Aslanzadeh J, Zheng X, Li H, *et al.* Prospective evaluation of rapid antigen tests for diagnosis of respiratory syncytial virus and human metapneumovirus infections. *J Clin Microbiol* 2008; 46: 1682–1685.
121. Doan Q, Enarson P, Kissoon N, *et al.* Rapid viral diagnosis for acute febrile respiratory illness in children in the Emergency Department. *Cochrane Database Syst Rev* 2009; 4: CD006452.
122. Centers for Disease Control and Prevention. 2015. RSV. For Healthcare Professionals. www.cdc.gov/rsv/clinical/ Date last accessed: February 18, 2016. Date last updated: April 20, 2015.
123. Casiano-Colón AE, Hulbert BB, Mayer TK, *et al.* Lack of sensitivity of rapid antigen tests for the diagnosis of respiratory syncytial virus infection in adults. *J Clin Virol* 2003; 28: 169–174.
124. Chartrand C, Tremblay N, Renaud C, *et al.* Diagnostic accuracy of rapid antigen detection tests for respiratory syncytial virus infection: systematic review and meta-analysis. *J Clin Microbiol* 2015; 53: 3738–3749.
125. Liao RS, Tomalty LL, Majury A, *et al.* Comparison of viral isolation and multiplex real-time reverse transcription-PCR for confirmation of respiratory syncytial virus and influenza virus detection by antigen immunoassays. *J Clin Microbiol* 2009; 47: 527–532.
126. Weinberg GA, Erdman DD, Edwards KM, *et al.* Superiority of reverse-transcription polymerase chain reaction to conventional viral culture in the diagnosis of acute respiratory tract infections in children. *J Infect Dis* 2004; 189: 706–710.
127. Falsey AR, Criddle MC, Walsh EE. Detection of respiratory syncytial virus and human metapneumovirus by reverse transcription polymerase chain reaction in adults with and without respiratory illness. *J Clin Virol* 2006; 35: 46–50.
128. Puppe W, Weigl J, Gröndahl B, *et al.* Validation of a multiplex reverse transcriptase PCR ELISA for the detection of 19 respiratory tract pathogens. *Infection* 2013; 41: 77–91.
129. Zhang C, Xiao Y, Du J, *et al.* Application of multiplex PCR couple with MALDI-TOF analysis for simultaneous detection of 21 common respiratory viruses. *J Clin Microbiol* 2015; 53: 2549–2554.

130. García-Arroyo L, Prim N, Martí N, *et al.* Benefits and drawbacks of molecular techniques for diagnosis of viral respiratory infections. Experience with two multiplex PCR assays. *J Med Virol* 2016; 88: 45–50.
131. Choi S-H, Chung J-W, Kim HR. Clinical relevance of multiple respiratory virus detection in adult patients with acute respiratory illness. *J Clin Microbiol* 2015; 53: 1172–1177.
132. Ahluwalia G, Embree J, McNicol P, *et al.* Comparison of nasopharyngeal aspirate and nasopharyngeal swab specimens for respiratory syncytial virus diagnosis by cell culture, indirect immunofluorescence assay, and enzyme-linked immunosorbent assay. *J Clin Microbiol* 1987; 25: 763–767.
133. Lambert SB, Whiley DM, O'Neill NT, *et al.* Comparing nose–throat swabs and nasopharyngeal aspirates collected from children with symptoms for respiratory virus identification using real-time polymerase chain reaction. *Pediatrics* 2008; 122: e615–e620.
134. Heikkinen T, Marttila J, Salmi AA, *et al.* Nasal swab *versus* nasopharyngeal aspirate for isolation of respiratory viruses. *J Clin Microbiol* 2002; 40: 4337–4339.
135. Chan KH, Peiris JSM, Lim W, *et al.* Comparison of nasopharyngeal flocked swabs and aspirates for rapid diagnosis of respiratory viruses in children. *J Clin Virol* 2008; 42: 65–69.
136. Munywoki PK, Hamid F, Mutunga M, *et al.* Improved detection of respiratory viruses in pediatric outpatients with acute respiratory illness by real-time PCR using nasopharyngeal flocked swabs. *J Clin Microbiol* 2011; 49: 3365–3367.
137. Englund JA, Piedra PA, Jewell A, *et al.* Rapid diagnosis of respiratory syncytial virus infections in immunocompromised adults. *J Clin Microbiol* 1996; 34: 1649–1653.
138. National Institute for Health and Care Excellence. Bronchiolitis in children: diagnosis and management. www.nice.org.uk/guidance/ng9 Date last accessed: February 18, 2016. Date last updated: June 1, 2015.
139. Turner T, Wilkinson F, Harris C, *et al.* Evidence based guideline for the management of bronchiolitis. *Aust Fam Phys* 2008; 37: 6–13.
140. Lee FE-H, Walsh EE, Falsey AR. The effect of steroid use in hospitalized adults with respiratory syncytial virus-related illness. *Chest* 2011; 140: 1155–1161.
141. Simões EAF, DeVincenzo JP, Boeckh M, *et al.* Challenges and opportunities in developing respiratory syncytial virus therapeutics. *J Infect Dis* 2015; 211: Suppl. 1, S1–S20.
142. Weigt SS, Gregson AL, Deng JC, *et al.* Respiratory viral infections in hematopoietic stem cell and solid organ transplant recipients. *Semin Respir Crit Care Med* 2011; 32: 471–493.
143. Fuller H, Del Mar C. Immunoglobulin treatment for respiratory syncytial virus infection. *Cochrane Database Syst Rev* 2006; 4: CD004883.
144. Liu F, Ouyang J, Sharma AN, *et al.* Leukotriene inhibitors for bronchiolitis in infants and young children. *Cochrane Database Syst Rev* 2015; 3: CD010636.
145. Beigelman A, Mikols CL, Gunsten SP, *et al.* Azithromycin attenuates airway inflammation in a mouse model of viral bronchiolitis. *Respir Res* 2010; 11: 90.
146. Beigelman A, Isaacson-Schmid M, Sajol G, *et al.* Randomized trial to evaluate azithromycin's effects on serum and upper airway IL-8 levels and recurrent wheezing in infants with respiratory syncytial virus bronchiolitis. *J Allergy Clin Immunol* 2015; 135: 1171–1178.
147. Tahan F, Ozcan A, Koc N. Clarithromycin in the treatment of RSV bronchiolitis: a double-blind, randomised, placebo-controlled trial. *Eur Respir J* 2007; 29: 91–97.
148. DeVincenzo J, Lambkin-Williams R, Wilkinson T, *et al.* A randomized, double-blind, placebo-controlled study of an RNAi-based therapy directed against respiratory syncytial virus. *Proc Natl Acad Sci U S A* 2010; 107: 8800–8805.
149. Gottlieb J, Zamora MR, Hodges T, *et al.* ALN-RSV01 for prevention of bronchiolitis obliterans syndrome after respiratory syncytial virus infection in lung transplant recipients. *J Heart Lung Transplant* 2016; 35: 213–221.
150. DeVincenzo JP, Whitley RJ, Mackman RL, *et al.* Oral GS-5806 activity in a respiratory syncytial virus challenge study. *N Engl J Med* 2014; 371: 711–722.
151. DeVincenzo JP, McClure MW, Symons JA, *et al.* Activity of oral ALS-008176 in a respiratory syncytial virus challenge study. *N Engl J Med* 2015; 373: 2048–2058.
152. Jorquera PA, Anderson L, Tripp RA. Understanding respiratory syncytial virus (RSV) vaccine development and aspects of disease pathogenesis. *Expert Rev Vaccines* 2016; 15: 173–187.
153. Alexander-Miller MA. Vaccines against respiratory viral pathogens for use in neonates: opportunities and challenges. *J Immunol* 2014; 193: 5363–5369.
154. Kim HW, Canchola JG, Brandt CD, *et al.* Respiratory syncytial virus disease in infants despite prior administration of antigenic inactivated vaccine. *Am J Epidemiol* 1969; 89: 422–434.
155. Guvenel AK, Chiu C, Openshaw PJ. Current concepts and progress in RSV vaccine development. *Expert Rev Vaccines* 2014; 13: 333–344.
156. Gonzalez IM, Karron RA, Eichelberger M, *et al.* Evaluation of the live attenuated *cpts* 248/404 RSV vaccine in combination with a subunit RSV vaccine (PFP-2) in healthy young and older adults. *Vaccine* 2000; 18: 1763–1772.

157. The IMpact-RSV Study Group. Palivizumab, a humanized respiratory syncytial virus monoclonal antibody, reduces hospitalization from respiratory syncytial virus infection in high-risk infants. *Pediatrics* 1998; 102: 531–537.
158. Committee on Infectious Diseases and Bronchiolitis Guidelines. Updated guidance for palivizumab prophylaxis among infants and young children at increased risk of hospitalization for respiratory syncytial virus infection. *Pediatrics* 2014; 134: 415–420.

Support statement: EU FP7 PREPARE grant 602525; Wellcome Programme: Immune regulation in viral lung disease, 16 November 2009–15 November 2015 (P25092: 087805/Z/08/Z) National Institute of Healthcare Research (NIHR) Imperial College Healthcare Trust Biomedical Research Centre (BRC) grant P45058; NIHR Senior Investigator Award; and NIHR Health Protection Research Unit (NIHR HPRU) in Respiratory Infections at Imperial College London in partnership with Public Health England. The views expressed are those of the author (s) and are not necessarily those of the National Health Service, the NIHR, the Department of Health or Public Health England.

Disclosures: P.J.M. Openshaw reports grants from the Wellcome Trust Translational Award, outside the submitted work.

Chapter 6

Human rhinoviruses

Stephen Oo[1,2] and Peter Le Souef[1,2]

Rhinovirus (RV) PCR techniques have been refined in the past two decades. They have redefined the epidemiology of this virus and have resulted in the discovery of a third species, *Rhinovirus C* (RV-C), in addition to the species *Rhinovirus A* (RV-A) and *Rhinovirus B* (RV-B). Alterations in the RV genome have allowed insight into the evolution of RV strains. The surface structure and cellular receptors differ among RV species, particularly for RV-C. For RV-C, the differences compared with RV-A and RV-B in these attributes suggest that the host immune responses against this virus may also differ from the other species. RV has long been associated with acute asthma, and RV-C has been found to be more common in acute severe asthma in children. The discovery of CDHR3 as the probable receptor for RV-C opens the way for biological and mechanistic studies. Genome-wide association studies have identified childhood asthma risk genes, namely *GSMDB*, *ORMDL3* and *CDHR3*. The demonstration of RV relevance to these genes supports previous theories about RV in asthma pathogenesis.

Rhinovirus (RV), as its name suggests, has been associated primarily with upper respiratory tract infections and is the most common virus detected (30–50%) during "common colds" [1]. This led to earlier misconceptions that RV causes a relatively benign illness. In the last two decades, a resurgence of interest has been spurred first from the discovery of its relevance in asthma and asthma exacerbations [2], particularly in more severe disease in both children and adults [3, 4], and secondly, by the development of PCR techniques for RV identification, which have increased accuracy and reduced labour and costs, and thus have made accessibility much easier. The most extraordinary outcome of PCR identification has been the discovery of a new species of RV, named *Rhinovirus C* (RV-C).

The discovery of RV-C has necessitated a re-evaluation of past RV research. Thus, this chapter aims to provide a semi-historical account to give context to current research directions and explain the ideological shifts in the classification, structure, genetics, epidemiology and clinical disease of RV.

Nomenclature and classification

The first RV was discovered some 60 years ago by Pelon *et al.* [5] and Price [6] who, working independently, reported the isolation of a new virus now designated RV-A1.

[1]School of Paediatrics & Child Health, Faculty of Medicine Dentistry and Health Sciences, University of Western Australia, Perth, Australia. [2]Respiratory and Sleep Dept, Princess Margaret Hospital, Perth, Australia.

Correspondence: Stephen Oo, Respiratory and Sleep Dept, Princess Margaret Hospital, Roberts Road, Subiaco, Perth, Western Australia, 6008, Australia. E-mail: stephen.oo@health.wa.gov.au

 Print ISBN: 978-1-84984-069-9. Online ISBN: 978-1-84984-070-5. Print ISSN: 2312-508X. Online ISSN: 2312-5098.

Through serotyping and immunogenic cross-reactivity, further RV species were identified and sequentially numbered, with 55 strains identified by 1967, before being expanded to 89 by 1971 and finally to 100 in 1987 [7]. Prototypes of these 101 serotypes were stored by the American Type Culture Collection; however, recent interrogation has revealed there to be only 98 individual serotypes. Over the years, these have been classified and grouped in multiple ways based on structure, function, drug response and genotyping.

RV is classified as a member of the family *Picornaviridae*, which includes 29 genera, including viruses such as poliovirus and enteroviruses. Originally, enteroviruses and RVs were classified in separate genera on the basis of diverging clinical features. Enteroviruses, as the name suggests, produce more gastrointestinal symptoms, largely because they are acid stable at pH 3 and can transit the stomach intact, as opposed to RVs, which are acid labile at pH <6. Acid lability was used to divide enteroviruses and RVs until the previously named RV-87 was revealed to be an acid-labile virus, enterovirus D [8, 9]. This, in combination with strong nucleotide sequence similarities, eventually led to RV species being reclassified by the International Committee on Taxonomy of Viruses into the genus *Enterovirus* in 2008 [10]. In 2012, all species of the genus *Enterovirus* were renamed to drop the host designations and so the formerly named "human rhinovirus" became just rhinovirus (RV).

The species *Rhinovirus A* (RV-A) and *Rhinovirus B* (RV-B) were assigned in 1999 based on clear genotypic differences between the two groups [11]. In 2006, following wider utilisation of PCR methods for RV typing, reports of a possible new species of RV emerged from Queensland [12], New York [13] and Switzerland [14]. Further sequencing performed by the Queensland group [15] confirmed that this species was similar but genotypically distinct from RV-A. Confirmation followed from cohorts in Hong Kong [16], California [17] and Germany [18]. In 2010, these strains were designated as a new third species, RV-C [19]. RV-C has been estimated to be in existence for >250 years, and many strains are widely co-circulating throughout the world [20]. RV discovery is still ongoing, but there are currently 80 strains of RV-A, 32 strains of RV-B and 55 strains of RV-C [21].

RV genetics

RVs, like all members of the family *Picornaviridiae*, are single-stranded, positive-sense RNA viruses. The genome structure is similar in all members of the family, with three protein-coding regions, P1, P2 and P3, enclosed at each end by an untranslated region (UTR) (figure 1). The P1 region encodes the four structural capsid proteins, which are numerically

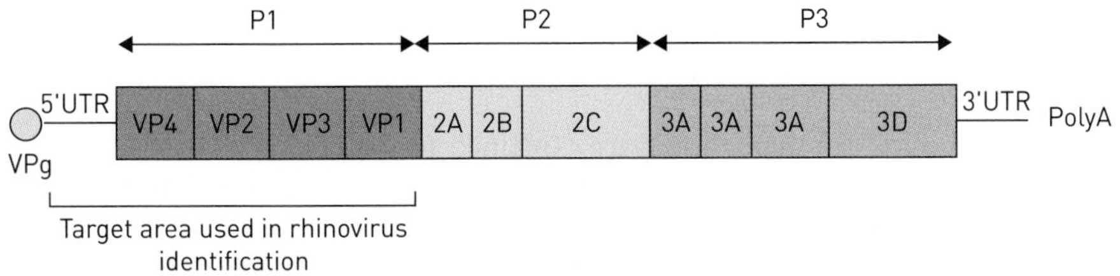

Figure 1. Typical genome structure of picornaviruses. P1 area encompasses the genes encoding capsid viral protein (VP) 1–4; P2 and P3 areas encode genes important in replication. The P1 and 5′ untranslated region (UTR) gene regions are most reliably utilised for rhinovirus detection and sequencing. VPg: viral protein genome-linked.

named viral protein 1 (VP1) to VP4. The P2 and P3 regions encode proteins important for virus replication.

RVs were first fully sequenced in 1984, commencing with serotype RV-B14 [22], and full sequencing of all of the 101 classic serotypes was completed in 2009 [23]. With newer RVs increasingly being classified based on genotyping, the terminology has shifted away from serotype to "type" or "strain", and the latter term will be used in this article. The original serotyping classifications have also come into question, with RV-A8 and RV-A95 showing a near-identical genotype, as well as serotype cross-reactivity [24]. The same has been shown for strains RV-A29/RV-A44 and RV-A54/RV-A98, and has led to a move to abolish serotypes A95, A44 and A98, thus leaving 98 classic serotypes [24].

Much has been published in the last 10 years regarding the methodology of RV PCR detection and sequencing. Three excellent reviews have been published previously on this subject [24–26]. Here, we will provide a brief overview.

The primers used in RV sequencing are not standardised and, although this is still an evolving subject, efforst are being made to make both techniques and primers more standardised. In detecting all RV strains, published primers do not perform in the same way, and no single pair accurately detects all RV strains [27]. Hence, for accurate detection, more than one PCR is required. Common methods use primers that generally target a combination of the 5′UTR and regions corresponding to capsid proteins VP4/VP2 or VP1.

Generally, the initial detection of RV occurs using universal diagnostic primers that target highly conserved motifs in the 5′UTR, as these tend to be the most sensitive [25, 28]. This region can be used for species and strain assignment with reasonable accuracy [28, 29], but, due to recombination events downstream, the results can be less reliable [26, 30]. This method does give a false-positive rate of ~5%, where human genomic DNA from chromosome 6 can be amplified and gives an amplicon of a similar size to that of RV [25–27]. Furthermore, different commercial assays utilise primer probes that target the same sequence but give repeatable but diverging results on the same samples, suggesting problems with probe hybridisation [31]. This may explain the substantially lower RV detection rates in some studies.

Sequencing of the VP4/VP2 or VP1 regions, respectively, gives unambiguous RV species and strain classification [26]. However, these regions are more variable and impede the design of universal primers. VP4/VP2 has been used in a large number of studies, mainly due to its shorter read length, greater sequence conservation and the wider library of known sequences available in GenBank [24]. The proposed criteria for the classification of a new strain of RV is >10% nucleotide divergence of VP4/VP2 from the nearest related strain, and >12–13% nucleotide divergence in VP1 [24, 25].

Diversity in RV species genotype is in part explained by an error-prone RNA polymerase, common in members of the family *Picornaviridae*, which allows accumulation of nucleotide mutations over a short time period. In RVs, there is an estimated error rate of 3.4×10^{-4} errors per nucleotide per cycle of replication *in vivo* and 8.4×10^{-4} *in vitro* [32]. This is a similar nucleotide error rate to other members of the family *Picornaviridae* [33, 34]. Hot spots for errors imply selection pressures for certain regions, and these exist primarily in the external capsid proteins VP1, VP2 and VP3, and in the non-structural genes encoding the 3C protease, 3D polymerase and 2C protein [32, 35]. Cold spots were found in the genes encoding VP4, 2A, 2B, 3A, 3B and 3D [32]. Overall, RV-C strains exhibit a greater genetic diversity when compared with RV-A and RV-B strains [36].

Recombination events have also affected RV strain diversity, with the majority involving the 5′UTR region [23, 28]. With the availability of full-genome sequences, a Bayesian approach was utilised recently to characterise the evolution of RV genomes and to fully evaluate recombination events and produce an accurate phylogenetic tree of RV strains (figure 2) [37]. This divided RV-C into two distinct groups, C1 and C2, with C2 formed by recombination events with RV-A mostly at the 5′UTR. RV-A clusters into four genotypically distinct populations, whereas all RV-B strains are genotypically similar. This segregation is useful, as genetic clustering translates into similar structure and function, and can help grouping in future epidemiological studies to investigate differences beyond species variations.

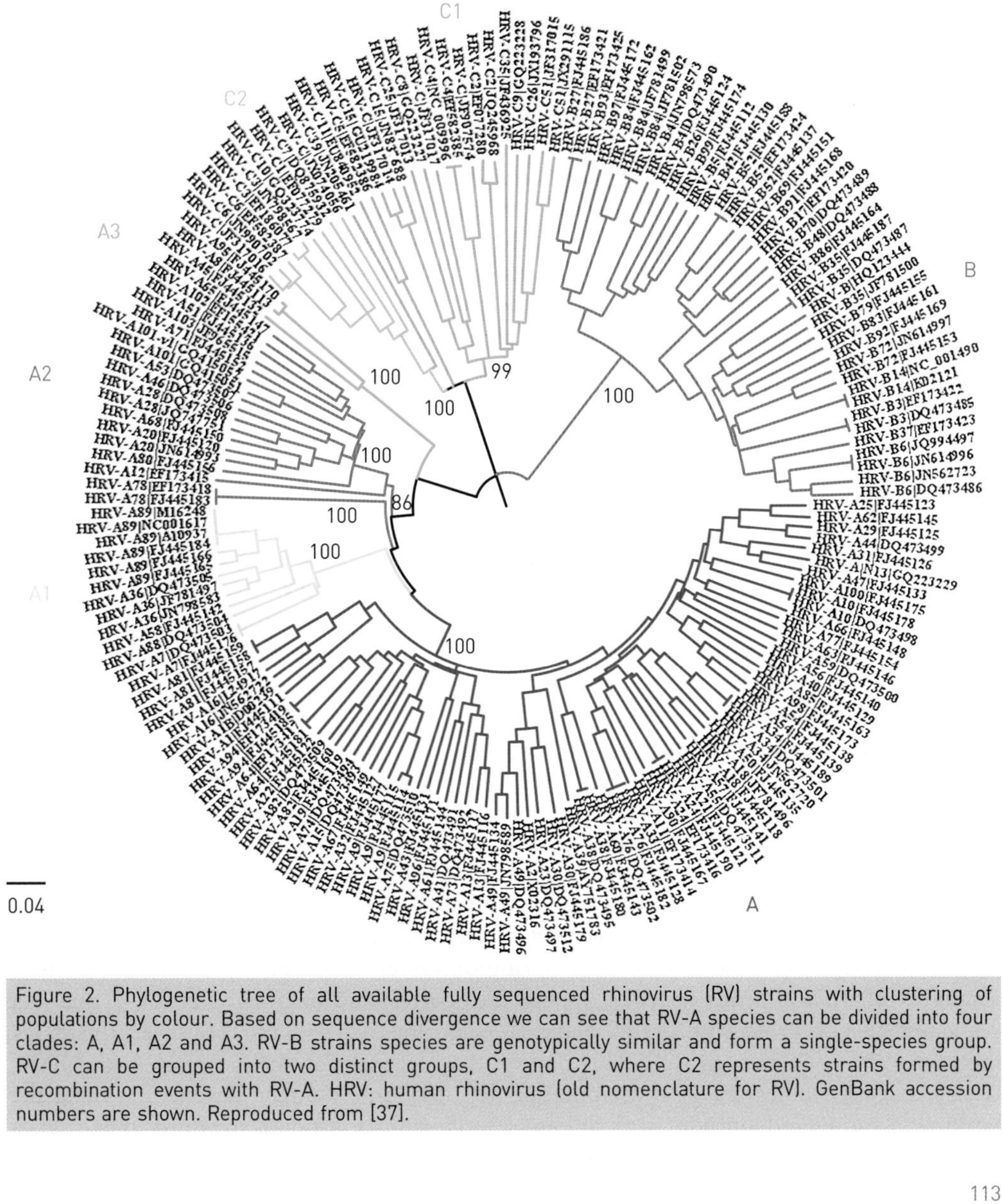

Figure 2. Phylogenetic tree of all available fully sequenced rhinovirus (RV) strains with clustering of populations by colour. Based on sequence divergence we can see that RV-A species can be divided into four clades: A, A1, A2 and A3. RV-B strains species are genotypically similar and form a single-species group. RV-C can be grouped into two distinct groups, C1 and C2, where C2 represents strains formed by recombination events with RV-A. HRV: human rhinovirus (old nomenclature for RV). GenBank accession numbers are shown. Reproduced from [37].

Clinical disease

Following RV PCR development, a large number of studies have been published in multiple clinical settings [38–42]. This has meant better characterisation of the role of RV in the setting of upper respiratory tract infections ("cold and flu"-like symptoms and pharyngitis), lower respiratory tract infections (croup, asthma, bronchiolitis and pneumonia) and, less commonly, febrile syndromes, apnoea, sepsis, rashes, otitis media, gastroenteritis and possibly even meningitis [43, 44].

Acute respiratory infections

Although RV is known as a common cause of upper respiratory tract infections, it has been recognised as a cause of lower respiratory tract infections since the 1960s [45]. PCR has allowed more accurate characterisation of these infections and a description of circulating strains. Unlike influenza where there is usually dominance of a particular strain at one time, multiple RV strains co-circulate throughout the community, and dominance of a single strain is seen only in groups of people co-habiting [46].

Transmission is thought to require close contact and spread from nasal secretions. While aerosol spread is possible, hand contact with nasal secretions is thought to be the most efficient method of transmission [47]. The rate of infection in healthy children is approximately one infection every 1–2 months, and half of these infections are asymptomatic [48]. The rate of infection in healthy adults has not been studied longitudinally, other than in the context of infected households. RV infection in adults is likely to be less frequent and often asymptomatic, infections usually being transmitted by the youngest child [38]. Infants and young children are particularly susceptible, and RVs are detected in approximately 50% of upper and 40% of lower respiratory tract infections [49].

In experimental inoculation of healthy adult volunteers, RV infection results in significant coryzal symptoms at 16 h post-inoculation, with a peak at 48 h, and declines to baseline levels by day 5 [50]. Viral titres are detectable at 10 h and peak at 48 h [50]. Longitudinal studies involving weekly aspirates in children have shown that RV RNA in children can be detected from a few days up to a week preceding clinical symptoms. In most cases, viral RNA becomes undetectable 2–3 weeks after the onset of symptoms up to a maximum of 5 weeks [51, 52]. Patients with symptoms extending beyond 5 weeks will almost always have a second virus, as the same RV strain has not been detected in the same patient after 5 weeks unless immunodeficiency is present [28].

RV has classically been described in temperate countries as having circulation throughout the year but with peaks in autumn and spring. This is in contrast to RSV and influenza virus, which tend to have strong peaks in winter [53–55]. Peaks in RV infection appear to correspond to children returning to school, and this corresponds to peak asthma periods [56, 57]. Species differences for these peaks have also been explored, and whether RV-A and RV-C is more common in autumn, spring or winter varies among studies [39, 58]. In a number of studies, peaks of RV-A appeared to correspond to troughs in RV-C and vice versa; and this occurred with overall biannual peaks for each [59, 60]. However, this is not the case in all countries [61, 62]. This pattern may account for skews in RV-A and RV-C relative rates if studies are of short duration [63, 64]. Interestingly, despite RV incidence peaking in spring and autumn, peak disease severity still corresponds to winter [65].

Given the inability to culture RV-C for biological experiments until recently, a greater emphasis has been placed on epidemiological characterisation of this virus. To date, there have been almost 100 studies determining the proportion of RV species including RV-C, and so reasonable conclusions can now be drawn. In ARI presentations other than wheezing/asthma, RV-A is the most common RV species detected, and this is especially true in community studies [58, 66, 67]. RV-C is the second most common species detected, with RV-B generally detected infrequently. In terms of disease duration, a recent community study of young children demonstrated shorter virus shedding times in those with RV-C (mean 7 days), compared with RV-A (mean 14 days, p=0.002) and RV-B (mean 14 days, p=0.012) [68].

Gastroenteritis and meningitis

The potential for RV to cause symptoms other than respiratory infections is a relatively new discovery. The acid lability of RVs, as discussed above, made gastrointestinal infections seem unlikely; however, RV RNA for all three species has been detected in 10% of stool cultures [44]. High viral RNA loads in the stool suggested that RV causes active gastrointestinal infection rather than being detected as a result of swallowed respiratory secretions [44]. Given the potential to produce similar clinical symptoms to enteroviruses, the same study analysed 1500 cerebrospinal fluid samples but found only one that was positive for RV, making RV meningitis possible but an exceptionally rare occurrence. Of interest, there is recent documentation of a fatal case of bronchiolitis in a previously healthy infant with no comorbidities other than a history of recurrent bronchiolitis, where RV-C was detected in multiple post-mortem specimens including the cerebrospinal fluid [69].

Asthma and asthma exacerbations

An association between RV and asthma exacerbations has been known since the 1970s [70]. However, the strength of this association was not demonstrated clearly until 1995, when Johnston *et al.* [2], tracking asthmatic children longitudinally, showed that a virus could be detected in >80% of exacerbations, and about two-thirds were accounted for by RV. These findings have since been replicated in multiple studies investigating wheeze in children (table 1). Similar rates of RV detection are found during asthma exacerbations in adult patients [3].

A large body of literature supports the notion that RVs affect individuals with asthma in a more profound way than those without asthma. Those with asthma are more susceptible to RV, have more symptoms (including a larger reduction in lung function) and are more likely to become hospitalised as a result of infection [43, 79, 80].

It has long been debated whether childhood wheezing should be considered asthma, as the majority of children stop wheezing by 5–6 years of age [81]. Given that there is no agreed definition of asthma and that the majority of acute exacerbations of both childhood wheeze and adult asthma are driven by RV infection, it would make more sense to consider these as part of a spectrum of the same disease. Indeed, one possible explanation for the disappearance of wheeze as children age may be that the majority of RV strains are encountered by school age and, with improving immunity from prior exposures, wheezing exacerbations become less common.

In the setting of wheeze, the distribution of the three RV species appears to vary with disease severity and age. As discussed above, RV-A has far greater prevalence in the community; however, in children <10 years of age and hospitalised with asthma/wheeze, RV-C is the most common virus seen. A summary of all available studies published in the context of asthma and wheeze is presented in table 1. The table shows that, in community studies or in children presenting to hospital with minor wheeze, RV-A was usually the most common RV species [39]. However, in children presenting to hospital with moderate to severe wheeze, RV-C was not only the most common RV species identified but was also associated with more severe disease [4, 16, 67, 71]. In nearly all studies, RV-B was less frequent and less severe. Patients who were hospitalised with RV-C wheezing had a higher likelihood of rehospitalisation compared with infection by other viruses (risk ratio 6.82, $p=0.001$) [40]. Possible reasons why RV-C may diverge clinically from RV-A and RV-B are discussed below (see Viral pathogenesis).

Why RV causes wheeze is an important question, and a current research focus is on host responses between those who wheeze with RV infection and those who do not. The potential reasons why individuals with asthma are susceptible to RV will be discussed later in the context of immunobiology, allergy and genetics.

Exacerbation of other respiratory diseases

RV infections have been shown to provoke infections in other obstructive respiratory diseases including cystic fibrosis (CF) and COPD, but not to the same degree as in asthma. In CF, RV is the leading virus found in CF exacerbations (16% of all exacerbations), but tends to follow a more benign course, despite resulting in greater use of antibiotics [41]. During CF exacerbations, RV-A and RV-C are detected in equal proportions, with RV-B rarely detected [82]. Infection with either RV-C or RV-A2 subspecies confers the greatest risk of CF exacerbations [83]. In COPD, RV is the leading virus implicated in exacerbations (24% of all exacerbations) [42]. Experimental RV infection of COPD subjects induces neutrophilic airway inflammation, lower airway symptoms and airflow obstruction; a subdued IFN response to virus is also demonstrated [84].

Viral pathogenesis

RV structure and drug therapy

The viral and capsid structure of RV-A and RV-B has been well described since the 1980s, utilising crystallographic and electron microscopy techniques. A basic understanding of capsid structure is necessary to understand the function of RV drug therapy and the host adaptive immune response.

All picornaviruses are non-enveloped and have a similar icosahedral capsid structure (figure 3). The capsid is built from 60 copies each of four proteins, VP1, VP2, VP3 and VP4 (see figure 1). Each four-protein unit is referred to as a protomer. VP1–VP3 are larger and surface exposed compared with the internalised VP4 protein. These proteins tessellate to form an almost featureless capsid exterior, particularly in RVs. The lack of surface projections in part explains the success of RVs in evading an immune response. However, a host receptor binding site on the capsid surface is cleverly hidden within a canyon formed at the intersection of VP1, VP2 and VP3 (figure 3). Significant variation in canyon structure between serotypes accounts for some of the different immunogenicity profiles, and also helps explain the current inability to create a universal RV vaccine.

Table 1. Summary of studies that account for rhinovirus (RV) species in the context of asthma and wheeze, listed by cohort age

First author [ref.]	Age demographics	Setting	Geographical location	Study recruitment time period	Population group and n	RV detected n (%)	% of overall RV detected: RV-A	RV-B	RV-C	Untypable/ EV %	Sample method	RV detection method	Species typing method
Smuts [71]	Median 12.2 months	Asthma, community/ hospital children	Cape Town, South Africa	May 2004–Nov 2005	Acute wheeze, n=220, admitted 35%, ICU 2%	128 (58.2), n=71 typed	36.6	8.5	4.2	NR	Nasal swab	5′UTR	5′UTR, VP4/VP2
Renwick [18]	Mean 5 months, median 10 months, range 2 weeks–5 years	Asthma/wheeze, hospital children	Bad Kreuznach, Germany	2003–2006	Retrospective samples where virus not found in n=97 cases	41 (42.3)	19.5	7.3	**73.2**	NR	NPA	MassTag PCR	VP4/VP2
Lau [16]	RV patients: median 1 year, range 7 days–8 years	Asthma/wheeze, hospital children	Hong Kong, China	Nov 2004–Oct 2005	Hospital children (RV patients, mostly asthma and wheeze), n=203	26 (12.8)	19.2	0.0	**80.8**	NR	NPA	VP4	VP4
Peltola [63]	Median age with RV 1.7 years	Asthma/wheeze, hospital children	Turku, Finland	Sep–Nov 2005	Hospitalisations, 61% with wheeze, n=163	46 (28.2)	23.9	4.3	**30.4**	NR	Nasal swab	Multiplex PCR (5′UTR)	5′UTR
Cox [40]	Mean 2.6 years, SD 16.6 months, range <5 years	Asthma/wheeze, hospital children	Perth, Australia	Dec 2000–Nov 2010	Acute wheeze/ asthma exacerbation n=197	135 (68.5)	25.9	2.2	**60.0**	11.1	Nasal samples	5′UTR	5′UTR
Moreira [72]	Median 4 years, range <1 years	ARI including wheeze, community children	São Paulo, Brazil	Mar–Dec 2008	Children with ARI (46.7% RV wheezing), n=120	56 (47.5)	21.4	10.7	**58.9**	NR	Nasal washing	5′UTR and VP4/VP2	5′UTR and VP4/VP2
Arden [73]	Median 5.1 years	Asthma/wheeze, hospital children	Queensland, Australia	Mar 2005–2007	Asthma exacerbation n=78	41 (52.6)	39	0	**56.1**	4.9	NPA	5′UTR	5′UTR
Mak [74]	Mean±SD asthma 5.6±3.6 years, controls 5.4±3.8 years	Asthma/wheeze, hospital children	Hong Kong, China	Oct 2008-Mar 2009	Asthma exacerbation n=128	107 (83.6)	17.8	0.0	**82.2**	NR	NPA	5′UTR	VP4/VP2
					Inpatient control, n=192	63 (32.8)	36.5	6.3	**57.1**	NR			
Bizzintino [4]	Mean±SD 6.4±3.3 years, range 2–16 years	Asthma/wheeze, hospital children	Perth, Australia	2002–2011	Acute wheeze/ asthma exacerbation n=128	112 (87.5)	30.4	1.8	**67.9**	1.8	NPA or nasal swabs	5′UTR	5′UTR
Olenec [64]	Mean 6.5 years, range 6–8 years	Asthma, community children	Madison, WI, USA	Only Apr and Sept 2006–2008	Asthmatics: weekly samples over 5 weeks, n=42 patients, n=501 samples	169 (33.7)	33	35	24	8	Nasal lavage	Respiratory multicode assay	5′UTR

Continued

Table 1. Continued

First author [ref.]	Age demographics	Setting	Geographical location	Study recruitment time period	Population group and n	RV detected n (%)	% of overall RV detected			Untypable/ EV %	Sample method	RV detection method	Species typing method
							RV-A	RV-B	RV-C				
Soto-Quiros [75]	Mean acute wheeze 8.8 years, stable asthma 9.1 years, controls 9.4 years, range 7–12 years	Asthma, community/ hospital children	San Jose, Costa Rica	Feb 2009 and Oct 2009	Acute wheeze, n=96	61 (63.5)	24.6	1.6	**75.4**	NR	Nasal wash	5′UTR	VP4/VP2
					Stable asthma, n=64	8 (12.5)	25.0	25.0	**50.0**	NR			
					Controls, n = 126	17 (13.5)	47.1	17.6	35.3	NR			
Kennedy [76]	Mean wheeze 8.9 years, acute rhinitis 10.5 years, controls 11.8 years, range 4–18 years	Asthma/wheeze, hospital children	Charlottesville, VA, USA	NR	Wheezing, n=28	16 (57.1)	50	0	50	NR	Nasal wash	Multiplex PCR	5′UTR
					Acute rhinitis, n=32	18 (56.3)	59	6	35	NR			
					Controls, n=14	1 (7.1)	0	0	**100**	NR			
Khetsuriani [77]	Mean NR, >6 years 70–75%, range 2–17 years	Asthma/wheeze, hospital children	Atlanta, GA, USA	Mar 2003–Feb 2004	Asthma exacerbation n=65	39 (60)	38.5	2. 6	20.5	38.5	Nasopharyngeal swab	5′UTR	VP1
					Asthma stable, n=7	18 (18)	16.7	11.1	0	72.2			
Denlinger [3]	Mean for groups 24–29 years	Asthma, community/ hospital children	WI, USA	2005–2009	Prospective: viral ALRI, n=66 patients (52 allergic asthma, 14 no asthma)	50 (75.8)	50.0	22.0	20.0	8.0	Nasal lavage and sputum	Respiratory multicode assay	5′UTR
McCulloch [78]	Mean age 47 years, range 18–82 years	Asthma, hospital adults	Atlanta, GA, USA	Oct 2009–Apr 2010	Retrospective >18 years of RV specimens, n=95	95	41.1	8.4	26.3	10.5	Clinical samples	xTAG respiratory viral panel	VP4/VP2
Kistler [17]	NR	Asthma, community adults	CA, USA	Autumn 2001–Dec 2004	Viral sampling if ARI: asthma exacerbation n=21	10 (47.6)	50.0	40.0	10.0	NR	Nasal lavage	VP4/VP2 and Virochip microarray	VP4/VP2
					Asthma no exacerbation n=32	15 (46.9)	66.7	20.0	13.3				
					No asthma, n=29	12 (41.4)	66.7	16.7	16.7				

Where RV-C shows greater proportion compared with RV-A or RV-B, RV-C has been highlighted in bold. Note that RV-A is most common in community studies and adults, and RV-C is most common in children hospitalised with acute wheezing. RV detection and species typing refer to the genome target of PCR primers used, or the best description in the study. EV: enterovirus; NR: not reported; UTR: untranslated region; VP: viral protein; NPA: nasopharyngeal aspirate; ALRI: acute lower respiratory infection.

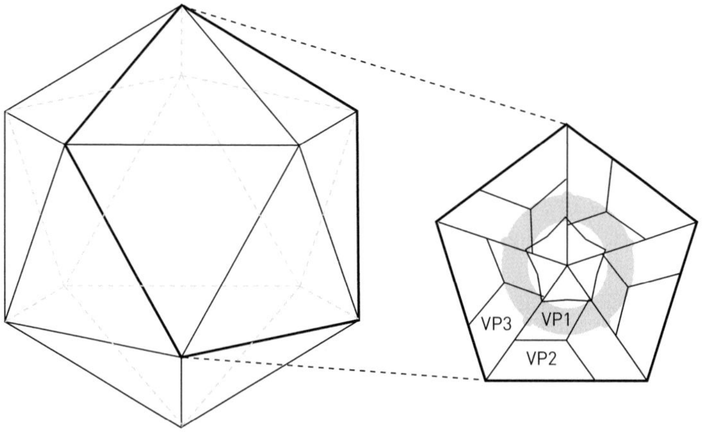

Figure 3. Schematic representation of the rhinovirus capsid overall icosahedral structure (left) and breakdown of the structure of the external capsid composed of tessellating viral protein (VP) units VP1–VP3, with VP4 being buried below the surface. The canyon region on the capsid surface (light grey shading) is one of the few features of the capsid surface and hides the binding site for host cellular receptors.

On binding to a host cell receptor, conformational changes occur in all proteins, but VP1 bends with a hinge-like action to allow VP1 and VP4 to penetrate the host cell membrane and viral RNA to be expelled into the cell (figure 4). A pocket, seen on the canyon surface of VP1, is integral in allowing VP1 to bend; this pocket is often described as the "drug-binding pocket". Drugs that insert into this pocket inhibit the conformational change of VP1 and therefore prevent viral RNA expulsion. When the 98 historic RV-A and RV-B

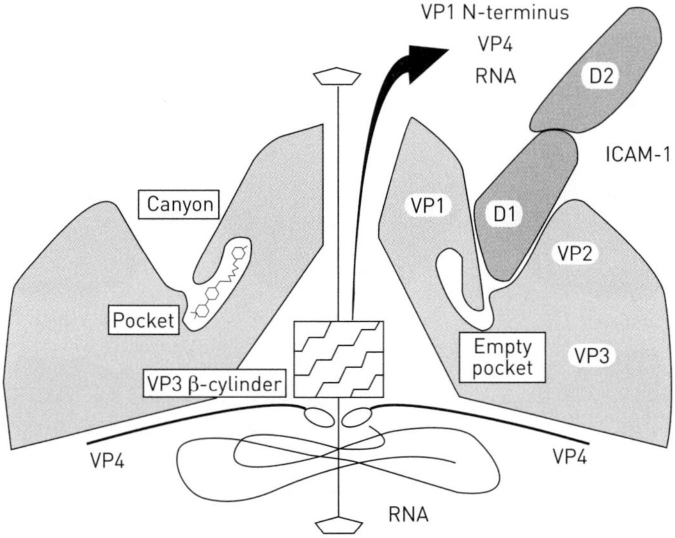

Figure 4. Cross-sectional representation of the rhinovirus capsid structure. On the left side, a pocket-binding drug sits in the pocket within the canyon, preventing conformational change in the event of intercellular adhesion molecule (ICAM)-1 binding. The right side demonstrates host cell ICAM-1 terminal domains D1 and D2 binding with a conformational change shown as a "hinge-like action" around the empty pocket, allowing opening of the central pore and extrusion of viral protein (VP)4 and VP1 to penetrate the host cell membrane and expulsion of viral RNA into the host cell. Reproduced and modified from [85] with permission from the publisher.

species were subjected to pocket-binding drugs, they divided into two experimental groups that corresponded roughly to species division [86]. Group 1 (all RV-B and six RV-A species) have a long narrow pocket and bind long-chain hydrophobic drugs (*e.g.* R61837). Group 2, predominantly comprising RV-A, have shorter, wider hydrophobic VP-1 pockets that bind a different class of molecule (*e.g.* WIN 51711). Drugs such as pleconaril (WIN 63843) bind the pocket in both groups and have been demonstrated to reduce viral load and the number of days of symptoms. However, 9% of clinical RV specimens demonstrate resistance to pleconaril [87], and these include strains of RV-C [88].

RV-C resistance to pleconaril may be caused by capsid surface structural changes to the canyon surface and the drug-binding pocket. The structure of RV-C is yet to be fully determined, but initial predictive modelling of protein sequences shows significant differences [89]. The structure of one strain, RV-C15, has been predicted using modelling software [90]. The model suggests striking differences in RV-C external capsid structure compared with other RV species (figure 5). RV-C is predicted to have a shallower canyon and flatter projected VP1 segments. These canyon structure differences may explain why pleconaril fails to inhibit RV-C15 replication [87].

Cellular receptor

Like all non-enveloped viruses, RV requires binding to a cellular receptor to gain entry into the host cell. There are at least three cellular receptors utilised by RV strains. RV strains that utilise intercellular adhesion molecule-1 (ICAM-1) are known as major group RVs, and include 85% of RV-A strains and 100% of RV-B strains. The remaining 10 serotypes of RV-A, which bind the low-density-lipoprotein receptor (LDLR), are termed the minor

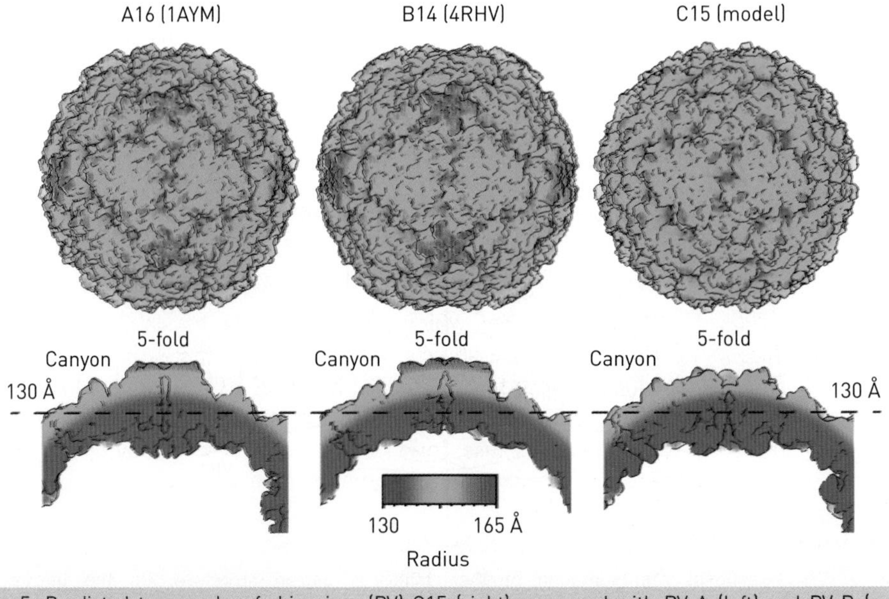

Figure 5. Predicted topography of rhinovirus (RV)-C15 (right) compared with RV-A (left) and RV-B (middle) strains. The upper diagrams show the overall capsid structure of the virus. The lower diagrams show a cross-sectional representation of the capsid through the 5-fold axes. Red represents elevations in surface projections and blue represents surface depressions. Note how the RV-C strain has substantially reduced surface projections and subsequently has a shallower canyon shape. Protein Data Bank numbers are shown in parentheses for RV-A16 and RV-B14. Reproduced and modified from [90] with permission from the publisher.

group [23]. There is some evidence to suggest that there are differences between the major and minor group RVs, with minor group RVs associated with more severe asthma exacerbations in adults [3].

RV-C is distinct in that it utilises neither LDLR nor ICAM-1. The most exciting recent revelation has been the identification of a probable cellular receptor for RV-C, namely CDHR3 [91]. By first identifying candidate receptor genes, these authors found, through systemic introduction of genes, that the *CDHR3* gene was the only gene that allowed the propagation of RV-C in HeLa cell lines. Not all candidate receptor genes that they identified have been explored, but their findings suggest that, even if CDHR3 is not the main receptor for RV-C, it is at least an important co-receptor. RV-C strains cannot be cultured in traditional cell culture media, and propagation of RV-C requires either mucosal or air–liquid interface cultures of fully differentiated cells, neither of which is likely to produce sufficient virus to enable biological or structural studies [87, 92, 93]. Nonetheless, this discovery opens the gateway to accessible RV-C for experimental purposes and biological characterisation.

At present, the exact function of CDHR3 is unknown, other than the fact that it is a member of a superfamily of cadherin molecules involved chiefly in transmembrane adhesion [91]. CDHR3 has been shown to be widely expressed in fetal and adult lungs [94]. Furthermore, a recently published genome-wide association study showed that single-nucleotide polymorphisms in *CDHR3* confer risk for the phenotype of recurrent severe exacerbations in young children [94]. Thus, the function of CDHR3 and potential changes induced by RV-C during asthma exacerbations are likely to be key areas of future research.

Knowledge of cellular receptor differences is also relevant to murine models of RV infection, as rodent ICAM-1 is different from human ICAM-1 [95]. For this reason, the majority of murine models of RV infection use RV-1B, a minor group RV that utilises LDLR. This is also part of the reason why few publications exist comparing differences in immune response and phenotype between minor and major group RV infections. The ability of rodents to be infected by RV-C is yet to be determined.

Cell infection and replication

RV was originally considered to be largely an upper-airways pathogen, as the ideal growth temperature in culture was traditionally found to be closer to that of the upper airways at around 33 °C, compared with lower airway, which are closer to a core temperature of 37 °C [96]. Papadopoulos *et al.* [96] have since shown that this is not the case for all classical RV-A and RV-B strains, and even those that replicated better at 33 °C replicated sufficiently to initiate infection. RV-C replicates equally well between 33 and 37 °C [93], suggesting that RV-C may be better suited to cause lower respiratory airways infections, and is therefore more likely to induce lower-airways inflammation and wheeze.

The efficiency of RV infections is remarkable. RV exhibits high infectivity with a small quantity of virus and, surprisingly, infects relatively few cells [97]. RV-infected cells demonstrate a healthy structure, and RV tends not to be cytopathic unless there are high doses of virus [97]. Minor group (LDLR) RV-A viruses appear to induce a greater cytopathic effect [98], and this may explain how these viruses cause a greater severity of symptoms in some people [3]. The overall lack of cellular damage observed during RV infections suggests that symptoms are related to upregulation of host responses to the virus.

Immunobiology

Host inflammation and inflammatory response

The host response to RV infection is complex. Following RV infection of epithelial cells, nuclear factor (NF)-κB intracellular signalling pathways are upregulated, causing a multifunctional response. This includes upregulation and expression of ICAM-1 and LDLR [99–101], which aid immune cell migration. However, by upregulating its own cellular receptors, RV demonstrates how it exploits the normal immune response. ICAM-1 induction has not been found by all researchers [98, 102], and one explanation for these apparent discrepancies is that RV binds ICAM-1 epitopes that are also used for antibody detection in these experiments. In addition, ICAM-1 expression is also induced by other T-helper 2 (Th2) cytokines commonly seen in asthma and allergy [103].

RV infection leading to NF-κB signalling also induces the release of an array of pro-inflammatory cytokines in the epithelium, many of which are also implicated in asthma and allergy. These include: granulocyte–macrophage colony-stimulating factor, a potent activator of eosinophil survival and adhesion molecule expression, with a role to play in eosinophil superoxide generation and degranulation [102, 104]; IL-8, a potent chemoattractant for neutrophils and IL-5 activated eosinophils [102, 105]; IL-6, a pleiotropic acute-phase reactant that is an attractant for neutrophils and later monocytes, and is crucial for T-cells and for B-cell differentiation [102, 106, 107]; IL-11, which has a role in airways hyperresponsiveness and B- and T-cell inflammation [108, 109]; eotaxins, which are chemoattractants for eosinophils [110]; and RANTES, an attractant for neutrophils, and which stimulates eosinophil degranulation [98, 111].

RV can also attach to airways macrophages and induces IL-1, IL-8 and macrophage inflammatory protein (MIP)-1α, IFN-γ, TNF-α and IFN-α [112, 113]. MIP-1α acts as a major chemokine for lymphocytes [114], and TNF-α and IFN-γ induce a Th1 response [115].

These pathways ultimately result in airways neutrophilia, increased numbers of T-cells and, to a varying extent, increased eosinophils [116, 117]. Similar cytokine and immune cell changes are seen in individuals with and without asthma. The key difference in individuals with asthma may be the balance between IL-5 and IFN-γ, as this appears to shape T-cell expression into Th1 or Th2 cells [118]. External stimulation of the cellular infiltrate is also important, as eosinophil activation and neutrophil degranulation correlate with changes in airways hyperresponsiveness [119, 120]. Furthermore, the severity of cold symptoms following RV infection is also closely related to the inflammatory response [121].

Following experimental RV infection of individuals with asthma or allergy, an acute neutrophilia can be observed within 48 h in nasal secretions, the lower airways and the blood. This correlates with nasal IL-8 and granulocyte colony-stimulating factor (G-CSF) [116, 118]. A transient decrease in blood lymphocytes is also observed [116]. Viral titres and symptoms correlated with IL-8 and G-CSF, showing an inflammatory response proportional to the degree of virus infection [118]. The ability of RV to induce airways neutrophilia is of particular relevance to asthma, as the cellular content of induced sputum is frequently used to categorise an "asthma airway phenotype" into neutrophilic, eosinophilic or mixed granulocytic, with the phenotype being used to determine the probable response to therapies such as the anti-IL-5 (anti-eosinophil pathway) drug mepolizumab [122]. However, a longitudinal study of asthmatic children demonstrated that the cellular content of induced sputum fluctuated enormously in individuals over a year, which the authors speculated was due to intermittent respiratory virus infections, especially RV [123].

H1-antihistamines have been shown to exert effects beyond the H1 histamine receptor, and external effects are hypothesised to converge on NF-κB pathways [124, 125]. Evidence for this is that H1-antihistamines have been shown to reduce ICAM-1 upregulation in RV infections [126–128]. However, in treating common colds, they demonstrate only limited short-term effects and make no long-term symptomatic differences [129]. Similarly, antihistamines have no demonstrable role in persistent asthma without the presence of allergic rhinitis [124]. However, they have not been explored in the context of asthma exacerbations, and may be a beneficial adjuvant to acute asthma therapy.

Innate immune response

NF-κB also upregulates IFN pathways, particularly type I (IFN-α and IFN-β) and type III (IFN-λ) IFN responses [130]. These are fundamental to innate immunity and trigger a wide response, including the induction of antiviral proteins and induction of chemokines both to attract natural killer and Th1 cells and to activate natural killer and cytotoxic T-cells [131]. In addition they also induce apoptosis signalling in virus-infected cells [132].

RV infection induces strong upregulation of type I and III IFNs [133]. IFN regulatory factor-7 is an integral component of type I IFN pathways and has been shown to be the main upregulated gene hub in paediatric asthma exacerbations, presumably in response to RV [134, 135]. Despite this, stimulation with RV in asthmatics has shown a deficient IFN-β response in human bronchial epithelial cells [101], and deficient IFN-α in peripheral blood mononuclear cells [131]. A deficiency in IFN-λ has similarly been demonstrated in asthmatic human bronchial epithelial cells [136]. However, a deficient type I and III IFN response was not demonstrated in all studies [137, 138], especially in individuals whose asthma was well controlled [139].

A possible explanation for these discrepancies may be that IFN defects in individuals with asthma are induced rather than being intrinsic, and a mouse model of allergic airways inflammation published recently showed that induction of Th2 inflammation by chronic airways inflammation could suppress type I and type III IFN responses [140]. Finally, in a TLR-7 knockout mouse that exhibited an impaired type I IFN response, infection with mouse pneumonia virus resulted in upregulation of Th2 cytokines and induction of phenotypic asthma airways changes, including airways hyperreactivity [141]. In addition, only TLR-7-deficient mice were able to be sensitised to the allergen. Thus, an intriguing possibility exists whereby the high Th2 inflammation seen in asthma suppresses the IFN response, increasing the likelihood of further virus stimulation, which feeds into further Th2 inflammation, feeding a cycle that ultimately subverts antiviral defences and favours virus propagation.

Antibody response

As discussed earlier, the surface structure of the RV capsid lacks epitope targets for antibodies. Antibodies generally develop to VP1 as the most surface-exposed region of the viral capsid. Following infection, secretory IgA appears after approximately 7 days; however, symptoms have usually subsided at this stage and IgA is not thought to contribute to virus clearance [142]. Much later, at 6–8 weeks, IgG antibodies form, and these remain for approximately 1 year [142, 143]. In healthy individuals, titres of strain-specific RV antibodies and high titres correlate with greater protection and reduced signs and symptoms to experimental RV infection [144].

Antibody induction to RV appears to be generally poor. In a pre-trial screen, none of 22 patients demonstrated any neutralising antibodies for RV-16, a major group RV-A [118]. Specific RV-C IgG_1 antibodies are low in both adults and children compared with those specific for RV-A and RV-B, and the majority of the total antibody response to RV-C is cross-reactive with RV-A [145]. This may reflect a greater structural diversity of epitopes for RV-C. Antibody responses to RV-A, RV-B and RV-C are unexpectedly elevated in the asthmatic group and in those with the most symptoms [143, 146]. The reasons for this are unclear, but potentially the existence of antibodies may contribute to an increased immune response in individuals with asthma, or perhaps antibodies do not target neutralising epitopes and therefore do not confer protection [143]. Overall, antibody responses appear to play a limited role in RV defence, and therefore the role of innate and epithelial defences may be more important.

Early-life exposure, allergy and asthma development

There is growing evidence of synergism between viruses, allergens and wheezing. Substantial wheezing risk has been described in individuals who tested positive for virus and had IgE antibody to allergen (OR 104.1, 95% CI 16.3–663.7) [147]. However, no specific viruses were discriminated in this study, and therefore whether this effect applies to specific or all respiratory viruses is a key question. RSV causes wheezing at a younger age, and initial studies have shown promise with regard to the possibility of allergy development, as it appears that, in rodents, RSV promotes IgE allergen responses [148]. However, prospective studies in humans have failed to show that RSV wheezing predisposes to atopy [149, 150]. In recent years, early RV infection has been shown to confer a greater risk for future wheeze. In an Australian birth cohort of children with atopic parents, risk of asthma at 5 years was only significant for those who wheezed earlier in life with RV (OR 2.9, p=0.02), compared with RSV (OR 2.1 p=0.3) [151]. Similarly, the US Childhood Origins of ASThma project (COAST) birth cohort showed that the risk of asthma at 6 years when wheezing in the first 3 years of life with RSV (OR 2.8) was less than those wheezing with RV (OR=9.8), while combination of RV and RSV did not confer that much of a greater risk (OR=10) [152]. This has been replicated by showing that the risk of asthma is higher in those who acquire non-RSV bronchiolitis, particularly RV bronchiolitis [153].

While these studies show a strong association, whether RV acts as a "canary in the mine" or has a role in asthma development is still uncertain. Given the known strong asthma and allergy associations, studies from the late 1980s sought to determine whether RV infection and allergen stimulation together showed any additive effects. It was demonstrated that RV inoculation of human subjects with allergic rhinitis not only induced airways hyperresponsiveness but also increased susceptibility to further airway obstruction following additional allergen provocation for up to 4 weeks after infection, and this effect was not found in non-atopic individuals [154]. Further work showed that RV and allergen challenge in atopic patients caused elevations in airway eosinophils, histamine and TNF-α for up to 28 days [155], as well as a systemic response with elevation of plasma histamine [156].

Two schools of thought have emerged: does RV damage the airways epithelium making it more susceptible to allergen in those who are susceptible, or are allergy pathways upregulated in the setting of RV? Given that RV causes less cytopathic airway damage than RSV, it seems more likely that the host response to RV is implicated.

Asthma genetics and RV

Further exploration of RV interaction with asthma risk genes shows great promise. As discussed above, the discovery of *CDHR3* polymorphisms that increase expression of CDHR3 is likely to have great relevance to the relationship between RV-C and wheeze. In addition, RV has recently been shown to upregulate known childhood asthma risk genes found on chromosome 17q21. The seminal paper by Moffat *et al.* [157] showed that gene polymorphisms at 17q21 were strongly associated with non-allergic childhood-onset asthma. These findings have been replicated in multiple populations, and four of the 15 genes in this region, namely *ORMDL3* (orosomucoid-like 3), *GSMDB* (gasdermin B), *IKZF3* (IKAROS family zinc finger 3) and *MED34* (mediator of RNA polymerase II transcription subunit 34), have been shown to be associated with childhood asthma [158]. Of these genes, expression of *ORMDL3* and *GSMDB* in peripheral blood mononuclear cells seems to be most associated with asthma risk [159]. In the US COAST birth cohort, gene sequence variants at 17q21 in conjunction with early-life RV wheezing showed the greatest risk for asthma (OR 26.1) [160]. These authors went on to show that white blood cells from those with 17q21 risk genes, when stimulated with RV, upregulated *ORMDL3* and *GSMDB* expression to a far greater extent; however, they specifically conceded that the study was underpowered to determine whether this relationship also applied to RSV [160], and whether these interactions are RV specific is, therefore, yet to be determined.

The exact role of GSMDB and ORMDL3 is unclear; however, ORMDL3 functions as a regulator of sphingolipid synthesis and this may have effects on bronchial reactivity. In addition, ORMDL3 is proposed to mediate endoplasmic reticulum-mediated calcium signalling, leading to cell proliferation, remodelling and inflammation, and potentially also enhances virus replication [161]. Less is known about GSMDB, but it may have a role in secretory pathways and stem cell proliferation in normal epithelium [160]. Given the high profile of these discoveries, characterisation of these regulator molecules is likely to emerge soon.

Conclusion

Evidence is mounting that the relationship between RV and asthma/wheeze/atopy may be more than just an association. RV is a specifically human virus that infects no other species, and its success is evident in the number of circulating strains at any given time. This success is due to the fact that it evades the human immune system while manipulating cells for replication with minimal damage, while the inflammation it induces further subverts innate antiviral defences. Thus, RV appears to have evolved the skills to manipulate a subgroup of humans, namely those with asthma and atopy, and in doing so may have found an ideal host.

References

1. Johnston SL, Sanderson G, Pattemore PK, *et al.* Use of polymerase chain reaction for diagnosis of picornavirus infection in subjects with and without respiratory symptoms. *J Clin Microbiol* 1993; 31: 111–117.

2. Johnston SL, Pattemore PK, Sanderson G, *et al.* Community study of role of viral infections in exacerbations of asthma in 9-11 year old children. *BMJ* 1995; 310: 1225–1229.
3. Denlinger LC, Sorkness RL, Lee W-MM, *et al.* Lower airway rhinovirus burden and the seasonal risk of asthma exacerbation. *Am J Respir Crit Care Med* 2011; 184: 1007–1014.
4. Bizzintino J, Lee W-M, Laing IA, *et al.* Association between human rhinovirus C and severity of acute asthma in children. *Eur Respir J* 2011; 37: 1037–1042.
5. Pelon W, Mogabgab WJ, Phillips IA, *et al.* A cytopathogenic agent isolated from naval recruits with mild respiratory illnesses. *Proc Soc Exp Biol Med* 1957; 94: 262–267.
6. Price WH. The isolation of a new virus associated with respiratory clinical disease in humans. *Proc Natl Acad Sci USA* 1956; 42: 892–896.
7. Hamparian VV, Colonno RJ, Cooney MK, *et al.* A collaborative report: rhinoviruses – extension of the numbering system from 89 to 100. *Virology* 1987; 159: 191–192.
8. Savolainen C, Blomqvist S, Mulders MN, *et al.* Genetic clustering of all 102 human rhinovirus prototype strains: serotype 87 is close to human enterovirus 70. *J Gen Virol* 2002; 83: 333–340.
9. Blomqvist S, Savolainen C, Råman L, *et al.* Human rhinovirus 87 and enterovirus 68 represent a unique serotype with rhinovirus and enterovirus features. *J Clin Microbiol* 2002; 40: 4218–4223.
10. Knowles NJ, Hovi T, Hyypiä T, *et al. Picornaviridae. In:* Virus Taxonomy: Classification and Nomenclature of Viruses. Ninth Report of the International Committee on Taxonomy of Viruses. San Diego, Elsevier, 2012; pp. 855–880.
11. Van Regenmortel MHV, Fauquet CM, Bishop DHL, *et al.*, eds. Virus Taxonomy: Classification and Nomenclature of Viruses. Seventh Report of the International Committee on Taxonomy of Viruses. San Diego, Academic Press, 2000.
12. Arden KE, McErlean P, Nissen MD, *et al.* Frequent detection of human rhinoviruses, paramyxoviruses, coronaviruses, and bocavirus during acute respiratory tract infections. *J Med Virol* 2006; 78: 1232–1240.
13. Lamson D, Renwick N, Kapoor V, *et al.* MassTag polymerase-chain-reaction detection of respiratory pathogens, including a new rhinovirus genotype, that caused influenza-like illness in New York State during 2004–2005. *J Infect Dis* 2006; 194: 1398–1402.
14. Kaiser L, Aubert J-D, Pache J-C, *et al.* Chronic rhinoviral infection in lung transplant recipients. *Am J Respir Crit Care Med* 2006; 174: 1392–1399.
15. McErlean P, Shackelton LA, Lambert SB, *et al.* Characterisation of a newly identified human rhinovirus, HRV-QPM, discovered in infants with bronchiolitis. *J Clin Virol* 2007; 39: 67–75.
16. Lau SK, Yip CC, Tsoi HW, *et al.* Clinical features and complete genome characterization of a distinct human rhinovirus (HRV) genetic cluster, probably representing a previously undetected HRV species, HRV-C, associated with acute respiratory illness in children. *J Clin Microbiol* 2007; 45: 3655–3664.
17. Kistler A, Avila PC, Rouskin S, *et al.* Pan-viral screening of respiratory tract infections in adults with and without asthma reveals unexpected human coronavirus and human rhinovirus diversity. *J Infect Dis* 2007; 196: 817–825.
18. Renwick N, Schweiger B, Kapoor V, *et al.* A recently identified rhinovirus genotype is associated with severe respiratory-tract infection in children in Germany. *J Infect Dis* 2007; 196: 1754–1760.
19. Carstens EB. Ratification vote on taxonomic proposals to the International Committee on Taxonomy of Viruses (2009). *Arch Virol* 2010; 155: 133–146.
20. Briese T, Renwick N, Venter M, *et al.* Global distribution of novel rhinovirus genotype. *Emerg Infect Dis* 2008; 14: 944–947.
21. The Picornavirus Pages. The Pirbright Institute, UK. www.picornaviridae.com/ Date last accessed: January 5, 2016. Date last updated: December 12, 2015.
22. Stanway G, Hughes PJ, Mountford RC, *et al.* The complete nucleotide sequence of a common cold virus: human rhinovirus 14. *Nucleic Acids Res* 1984; 12: 7859–7875.
23. Palmenberg AC, Spiro D, Kuzmickas R, *et al.* Sequencing and analyses of all known human rhinovirus genomes reveal structure and evolution. *Science* 2009; 324: 55–59.
24. McIntyre CL, Knowles NJ, Simmonds P. Proposals for the classification of human rhinovirus species A, B and C into genotypically assigned types. *J Gen Virol* 2013; 94: 1791–1806.
25. Bochkov YA, Gern JE. Clinical and molecular features of human rhinovirus C. *Microbes Infect* 2012; 14: 485–494.
26. Arden KE, Mackay IM. Newly identified human rhinoviruses: molecular methods heat up the cold viruses. *Rev Med Virol* 2010; 20: 156–176.
27. Faux CE, Arden KE, Lambert SB, *et al.* Usefulness of published PCR primers in detecting human rhinovirus infection. *Emerg Infect Dis* 2011; 17: 296–298.
28. Wisdom A, Kutkowska AE, McWilliam Leitch EC, *et al.* Genetics, recombination and clinical features of human rhinovirus species C (HRV-C) infections; interactions of HRV-C with other respiratory viruses. *PLoS One* 2009; 4: e8518.
29. Lee W-M, Grindle K, Pappas T, *et al.* High-throughput, sensitive, and accurate multiplex PCR-microsphere flow cytometry system for large-scale comprehensive detection of respiratory viruses. *J Clin Microbiol* 2007; 45: 2626–2634.

30. Savolainen-Kopra C, Blomqvist S, Smura T, *et al.* 5′ Noncoding region alone does not unequivocally determine genetic type of human rhinovirus strains. *J Clin Microbiol* 2009; 47: 1278–1280.
31. Dupouey J, Ninove L, Ferrier V, *et al.* Molecular detection of human rhinoviruses in respiratory samples: a comparison of Taqman probe-, SYBR Green I- and BOXTO-based real-time PCR assays. *Virol J* 2014; 11: 31.
32. Cordey S, Junier T, Gerlach D, *et al.* Rhinovirus genome evolution during experimental human infection. *PLoS One* 2010; 5: e10588.
33. Harvala H, Simmonds P. Human parechoviruses: biology, epidemiology and clinical significance. *J Clin Virol* 2009; 45: 1–9.
34. Drake JW. The distribution of rates of spontaneous mutation over viruses, prokaryotes, and eukaryotes. *Ann N Y Acad Sci* 1999; 870: 100–107.
35. Kistler AL, Webster DR, Rouskin S, *et al.* Genome-wide diversity and selective pressure in the human rhinovirus. *Virol J* 2007; 4: 40.
36. Miller EK, Williams JV, Gebretsadik T, *et al.* Host and viral factors associated with severity of human rhinovirus-associated infant respiratory tract illness. *J Allergy Clin Immunol* 2011; 127: 883–891.
37. Waman VP, Kolekar PS, Kale MM, *et al.* Population structure and evolution of rhinoviruses. *PLoS One* 2014; 9: e88981.
38. Peltola V, Waris M, Osterback R, *et al.* Clinical effects of rhinovirus infections. *J Clin Virol* 2008; 43: 411–414.
39. Linder JE, Kraft DC, Mohamed Y, *et al.* Human rhinovirus C: age, season, and lower respiratory illness over the past 3 decades. *J Allergy Clin Immunol* 2013; 131: 69–77.e1–6.
40. Cox DW, Bizzintino J, Ferrari G, *et al.* Human rhinovirus species C infection in young children with acute wheeze is associated with increased acute respiratory hospital admissions. *Am J Respir Crit Care Med* 2013; 188: 1358–1364.
41. Smyth AR, Smyth RL, Tong CY, *et al.* Effect of respiratory virus infections including rhinovirus on clinical status in cystic fibrosis. *Arch Dis Child* 1995; 73: 117–120.
42. McManus TE, Marley A-M, Baxter N, *et al.* Respiratory viral infection in exacerbations of COPD. *Respir Med* 2008; 102: 1575–1580.
43. Miller EK, Lu X, Erdman DD, *et al.* Rhinovirus-associated hospitalizations in young children. *J Infect Dis* 2007; 195: 773–781.
44. Harvala H, McIntyre CL, McLeish NJ, *et al.* High detection frequency and viral loads of human rhinovirus species A to C in fecal samples; diagnostic and clinical implications. *J Med Virol* 2012; 84: 536–542.
45. Cherry JD, Diddams JA, Dick EC. Rhinovirus infections in hospitalized children. Provocative bacterial interrelationships. *Arch Environ Health* 1967; 14: 390–396.
46. Mubareka S, Louie L, Wong H, *et al.* Co-circulation of multiple genotypes of human rhinovirus during a large outbreak of respiratory illness in a veterans' long-term care home. *J Clin Virol* 2013; 58: 455–460.
47. Turner RB, Fuls JL, Rodgers ND, *et al.* A randomized trial of the efficacy of hand disinfection for prevention of rhinovirus infection. *Clin Infect Dis* 2012; 54: 1422–1426.
48. Lee W-M, Lemanske RF, Evans MD, *et al.* Human rhinovirus species and season of infection determine illness severity. *Am J Respir Crit Care Med* 2012; 186: 886–891.
49. Kusel MMH, de Klerk NH, Holt PG, *et al.* Role of respiratory viruses in acute upper and lower respiratory tract illness in the first year of life: a birth cohort study. *Pediatr Infect Dis J* 2006; 25: 680–686.
50. Harris JM II, Gwaltney JM Jr. Incubation periods of experimental rhinovirus infection and illness. *Clin Infect Dis* 1996; 23: 1287–1290.
51. Winther B, Hayden FG, Hendley JO. Picornavirus infections in children diagnosed by RT-PCR during longitudinal surveillance with weekly sampling: association with symptomatic illness and effect of season. *J Med Virol* 2006; 78: 644–650.
52. Jartti T, Lehtinen P, Vuorinen T, *et al.* Persistence of rhinovirus and enterovirus RNA after acute respiratory illness in children. *J Med Virol* 2004; 72: 695–699.
53. Calvo C, García-García ML, Blanco C, *et al.* Role of rhinovirus in hospitalized infants with respiratory tract infections in Spain. *Pediatr Infect Dis J* 2007; 26: 904–908.
54. Johnston NW, Johnston SL, Duncan JM, *et al.* The September epidemic of asthma exacerbations in children: a search for etiology. *J Allergy Clin Immunol* 2005; 115: 132–138.
55. Johnston SL, Pattemore PK, Sanderson G, *et al.* The relationship between upper respiratory infections and hospital admissions for asthma: a time-trend analysis. *Am J Respir Crit Care Med* 1996; 154: 654–660.
56. Johnston NW, Johnston SL, Norman GR, *et al.* The September epidemic of asthma hospitalization: school children as disease vectors. *J Allergy Clin Immunol* 2006; 117: 557–562.
57. Tovey ER, Rawlinson WD. A modern miasma hypothesis and back-to-school asthma exacerbations. *Med Hypotheses* 2011; 76: 113–116.
58. Zeng SZ, Xiao NG, Xie Z-P, *et al.* Prevalence of human rhinovirus in children admitted to hospital with acute lower respiratory tract infections in Changsha, China. *J Med Virol* 2014; 86: 1983–1989.
59. Lu Q-B, Wo Y, Wang L-Y, *et al.* Molecular epidemiology of human rhinovirus in children with acute respiratory diseases in Chongqing, China. *Sci Rep* 2014; 4: 6686.

60. Kaida A, Kubo H, Takakura K, *et al.* Molecular epidemiology of human rhinovirus C in patients with acute respiratory tract infections in Osaka City, Japan. *Jpn J Infect Dis* 2011; 64: 488–492.
61. Onyango CO, Welch SR, Munywoki PK, *et al.* Molecular epidemiology of human rhinovirus infections in Kilifi, coastal Kenya. *J Med Virol* 2012; 84: 823–831.
62. Linsuwanon P, Payungporn S, Suwannakarn K, *et al.* Complete coding sequence characterization and comparative analysis of the putative novel human rhinovirus (HRV) species C and B. *Virol J* 2011; 8: 5.
63. Peltola V, Jartti T, Putto-Laurila A, *et al.* Rhinovirus infections in children: a retrospective and prospective hospital-based study. *J Med Virol* 2009; 81: 1831–1838.
64. Olenec JP, Kim WK, Lee W-M, *et al.* Weekly monitoring of children with asthma for infections and illness during common cold seasons. *J Allergy Clin Immunol* 2010; 125: 1001–1006.
65. Lau SKP, Yip CCY, Lin AWC, *et al.* Clinical and molecular epidemiology of human rhinovirus C in children and adults in Hong Kong reveals a possible distinct human rhinovirus C subgroup. *J Infect Dis* 2009; 200: 1096–1103.
66. Wisdom A, Leitch ECM, Gaunt E, *et al.* Screening respiratory samples for detection of human rhinoviruses (HRVs) and enteroviruses: comprehensive VP4-VP2 typing reveals high incidence and genetic diversity of HRV species C. *J Clin Microbiol* 2009; 47: 3958–3967.
67. Miller EK, Khuri-Bulos N, Williams JV, *et al.* Human rhinovirus C associated with wheezing in hospitalised children in the Middle East. *J Clin Virol* 2009; 46: 85–89.
68. Principi N, Zampiero A, Gambino M, *et al.* Prospective evaluation of rhinovirus infection in healthy young children. *J Clin Virol* 2015; 66: 83–89.
69. Lupo J, Schuffenecker I, Morel-Baccard C, *et al.* Disseminated rhinovirus C8 infection with infectious virus in blood and fatal outcome in a child with repeated episodes of bronchiolitis. *J Clin Microbiol* 2015; 53: 1775–1777.
70. Gregg I. Viral infection and asthma. *Br Med J* 1972; 3: 824–825.
71. Smuts HE, Workman LJ, Zar HJ. Human rhinovirus infection in young African children with acute wheezing. *BMC Infect Dis* 2011; 11: 65.
72. Moreira LP, Kamikawa J, Watanabe ASA, *et al.* Frequency of human rhinovirus species in outpatient children with acute respiratory infections at primary care level in Brazil. *Pediatr Infect Dis J* 2011; 30: 612–614.
73. Arden KE, Chang AB, Lambert SB, *et al.* Newly identified respiratory viruses in children with asthma exacerbation not requiring admission to hospital. *J Med Virol* 2010; 82: 1458–1461.
74. Mak RKY, Tse LY, Lam WY, *et al.* Clinical spectrum of human rhinovirus infections in hospitalized Hong Kong children. *Pediatr Infect Dis J* 2011; 30: 749–753.
75. Soto-Quiros M, Avila L, Platts-Mills TAE, *et al.* High titers of IgE antibody to dust mite allergen and risk for wheezing among asthmatic children infected with rhinovirus. *J Allergy Clin Immunol* 2012; 129: 1499–1505.
76. Kennedy JL, Shaker M, McMeen V, *et al.* Comparison of viral load in individuals with and without asthma during infections with rhinovirus. *Am J Respir Crit Care Med* 2014; 189: 532–539.
77. Khetsuriani N, Lu X, Teague WG, *et al.* Novel human rhinoviruses and exacerbation of asthma in children. *Emerg Infect Dis* 2008; 14: 1793–1796.
78. McCulloch DJ, Sears MH, Jacob JT, *et al.* Severity of rhinovirus infection in hospitalized adults is unrelated to genotype. *Am J Clin Pathol* 2014; 142: 165–172.
79. Corne JM, Marshall C, Smith S, *et al.* Frequency, severity, and duration of rhinovirus infections in asthmatic and non-asthmatic individuals: a longitudinal cohort study. *Lancet* 2002; 359: 831–834.
80. DeMore JP, Weisshaar EH, Vrtis RF, *et al.* Similar colds in subjects with allergic asthma and nonatopic subjects after inoculation with rhinovirus-16. *J Allergy Clin Immunol* 2009; 124: 245–252, 252 e1-3.
81. Martinez FD, Wright AL, Taussig LM, *et al.* Asthma and wheezing in the first six years of life. The Group Health Medical Associates. *N Engl J Med* 1995; 332: 133–138.
82. Goffard A, Lambert V, Salleron J, *et al.* Virus and cystic fibrosis: rhinoviruses are associated with exacerbations in adult patients. *J Clin Virol* 2014; 60: 10–12.
83. de Almeida MB, Zerbinati RM, Tateno AF, *et al.* Rhinovirus C and respiratory exacerbations in children with cystic fibrosis. *Emerg Infect Dis* 2010; 16: 996–999.
84. Mallia P, Message SD, Gielen V, *et al.* Experimental rhinovirus infection as a human model of chronic obstructive pulmonary disease exacerbation. *Am J Respir Crit Care Med* 2011; 183: 734–742.
85. Kolatkar PR, Bella J, Olson NH, *et al.* Structural studies of two rhinovirus serotypes complexed with fragments of their cellular receptor. *EMBO J* 1999; 18: 6249–6259.
86. Andries K, Dewindt B, Snoeks J, *et al.* Two groups of rhinoviruses revealed by a panel of antiviral compounds present sequence divergence and differential pathogenicity. *J Virol* 1990; 64: 1117–1123.
87. Kaiser L, Crump CE, Hayden FG. In vitro activity of pleconaril and AG7088 against selected serotypes and clinical isolates of human rhinoviruses. *Antiviral Res* 2000; 47: 215–220.
88. Hao W, Bernard K, Patel N, *et al.* Infection and propagation of human rhinovirus C in human airway epithelial cells. *J Virol* 2012; 86: 13524–13532.
89. McErlean P, Shackelton LA, Andrews E, *et al.* Distinguishing molecular features and clinical characteristics of a putative new rhinovirus species, human rhinovirus C (HRV C). *PLoS One* 2008; 3: e1847.

90. Basta HA, Sgro J-YY, Palmenberg AC. Modeling of the human rhinovirus C capsid suggests a novel topography with insights on receptor preference and immunogenicity. *Virology* 2014; 448: 176–184.
91. Bochkov YA, Watters K, Ashraf S, *et al.* Cadherin-related family member 3, a childhood asthma susceptibility gene product, mediates rhinovirus C binding and replication. *Proc Natl Acad Sci USA* 2015; 112: 5485–5490.
92. Bochkov YA, Palmenberg AC, Lee WM, *et al.* Molecular modeling, organ culture and reverse genetics for a newly identified human rhinovirus C. *Nat Med* 2011; 17: 627–632.
93. Ashraf S, Brockman-Schneider R, Bochkov YA, *et al.* Biological characteristics and propagation of human rhinovirus-C in differentiated sinus epithelial cells. *Virology* 2013; 436: 143–149.
94. Bønnelykke K, Sleiman P, Nielsen K, *et al.* A genome-wide association study identifies CDHR3 as a susceptibility locus for early childhood asthma with severe exacerbations. *Nat Genet* 2014; 46: 51–55.
95. Bartlett NW, Walton RP, Edwards MR, *et al.* Mouse models of rhinovirus-induced disease and exacerbation of allergic airway inflammation. *Nat Med* 2008; 14: 199–204.
96. Papadopoulos NG, Sanderson G, Hunter J, *et al.* Rhinoviruses replicate effectively at lower airway temperatures. *J Med Virol* 1999; 58: 100–104.
97. Papadopoulos NG, Bates PJ, Bardin PG, *et al.* Rhinoviruses infect the lower airways. *J Infect Dis* 2000; 181: 1875–1884.
98. Schroth MK, Grimm E, Frindt P, *et al.* Rhinovirus replication causes RANTES production in primary bronchial epithelial cells. *Am J Respir Cell Mol Biol* 1999; 20: 1220–1228.
99. Papi A, Johnston SL. Rhinovirus infection induces expression of its own receptor intercellular adhesion molecule 1 (ICAM-1) *via* increased NF-κB-mediated transcription. *J Biol Chem* 1999; 274: 9707–9720.
100. Suzuki T, Yamaya M, Kamanaka M, *et al.* Type 2 rhinovirus infection of cultured human tracheal epithelial cells: role of LDL receptor. *Am J Physiol Lung Cell Mol Physiol* 2001; 280: L409–L420.
101. Wark PAB, Johnston SL, Bucchieri F, *et al.* Asthmatic bronchial epithelial cells have a deficient innate immune response to infection with rhinovirus. *J Exp Med* 2005; 201: 937–947.
102. Subauste MC, Jacoby DB, Richards SM, *et al.* Infection of a human respiratory epithelial cell line with rhinovirus. Induction of cytokine release and modulation of susceptibility to infection by cytokine exposure. *J Clin Invest* 1995; 96: 549–557.
103. Bianco A, Sethi SK, Allen JT, *et al.* Th2 cytokines exert a dominant influence on epithelial cell expression of the major group human rhinovirus receptor, ICAM-1. *Eur Respir J* 1998; 12: 619–626.
104. Nagata M, Sedgwick JB, Busse WW. Synergistic activation of eosinophil superoxide anion generation by VCAM-1 and GM-CSF. Involvement of tyrosine kinase and protein kinase C. *Int Arch Allergy Immunol* 1997; 114: Suppl. 1, 78–80.
105. Warringa RA, Schweizer RC, Maikoe T, *et al.* Modulation of eosinophil chemotaxis by interleukin-5. *Am J Respir Cell Mol Biol* 1992; 7: 631–636.
106. Zhu Z, Tang W, Ray A, *et al.* Rhinovirus stimulation of interleukin-6 *in vivo* and *in vitro*. Evidence for nuclear factor κB-dependent transcriptional activation. *J Clin Invest* 1996; 97: 421–430.
107. Scheller J, Chalaris A, Schmidt-Arras D, *et al.* The pro- and anti-inflammatory properties of the cytokine interleukin-6. *Biochim Biophys Acta* 2011; 1813: 878–888.
108. Tang W, Geba GP, Zheng T, *et al.* Targeted expression of IL-11 in the murine airway causes lymphocytic inflammation, bronchial remodeling, and airways obstruction. *J Clin Invest* 1996; 98: 2845–2853.
109. Einarsson O, Geba GP, Zhu Z, *et al.* Interleukin-11: stimulation *in vivo* and *in vitro* by respiratory viruses and induction of airways hyperresponsiveness. *J Clin Invest* 1996; 97: 915–924.
110. Papadopoulos NG, Papi A, Meyer J, *et al.* Rhinovirus infection up-regulates eotaxin and eotaxin-2 expression in bronchial epithelial cells. *Clin Exp Allergy* 2001; 31: 1060–1066.
111. Grissell TV, Powell H, Shafren DR, *et al.* Interleukin-10 gene expression in acute virus-induced asthma. *Am J Respir Crit Care Med* 2005; 172: 433–439.
112. Gern JE, Dick EC, Lee WM, *et al.* Rhinovirus enters but does not replicate inside monocytes and airway macrophages. *J Immunol* 1996; 156: 621–627.
113. Laza-Stanca V, Stanciu LA, Message SD, *et al.* Rhinovirus replication in human macrophages induces NF-κB-dependent tumor necrosis factor alpha production. *J Virol* 2006; 80: 8248–8258.
114. Schall TJ, Bacon K, Camp RD, *et al.* Human macrophage inflammatory protein alpha (MIP-1α) and MIP-1β chemokines attract distinct populations of lymphocytes. *J Exp Med* 1993; 177: 1821–1826.
115. van Benten IJ, KleinJan A, Neijens HJ, *et al.* Prolonged nasal eosinophilia in allergic patients after common cold. *Allergy* 2001; 56: 949–956.
116. Jarjour NN, Gern JE, Kelly EA, *et al.* The effect of an experimental rhinovirus 16 infection on bronchial lavage neutrophils. *J Allergy Clin Immunol* 2000; 105: 1169–1177.
117. Fraenkel DJ, Bardin PG, Sanderson G, *et al.* Lower airways inflammation during rhinovirus colds in normal and in asthmatic subjects. *Am J Respir Crit Care Med* 1995; 151: 879–886.
118. Gern JE, Vrtis R, Grindle KA, *et al.* Relationship of upper and lower airway cytokines to outcome of experimental rhinovirus infection. *Am J Respir Crit Care Med* 2000; 162: 2226–2231.

119. Grunberg K, Smits HH, Timmers MC, *et al.* Experimental rhinovirus 16 infection. Effects on cell differentials and soluble markers in sputum in asthmatic subjects. *Am J Respir Crit Care Med* 1997; 156: 609–616.
120. Wark PA, Johnston SLL, Moric I, *et al.* Neutrophil degranulation and cell lysis is associated with clinical severity in virus-induced asthma. *Eur Respir J* 2002; 19: 68–75.
121. Grunberg K, Timmers MC, Smits HH, *et al.* Effect of experimental rhinovirus 16 colds on airway hyperresponsiveness to histamine and interleukin-8 in nasal lavage in asthmatic subjects in vivo. *Clin Exp Allergy* 1997; 27: 36–45.
122. Nair P, Dasgupta A, Brightling CE, *et al.* How to diagnose and phenotype asthma. *Clin Chest Med* 2012; 33: 445–457.
123. Fleming L, Tsartsali L, Wilson N, *et al.* Sputum inflammatory phenotypes are not stable in children with asthma. *Thorax* 2012; 67: 675–681.
124. Simons FER. Advances in H1-antihistamines. *N Engl J Med* 2004; 351: 2203–2217.
125. Arnold R, Rihoux J, König W. Cetirizine counter-regulates interleukin-8 release from human epithelial cells (A549). *Clin Exp Allergy* 1999; 29: 1681–1691.
126. Jang YJ, Wang JH, Kim JS, *et al.* Levocetirizine inhibits rhinovirus-induced ICAM-1 and cytokine expression and viral replication in airway epithelial cells. *Antiviral Res* 2009; 81: 226–233.
127. Papi A, Papadopoulos NG, Stanciu LA, *et al.* Effect of desloratadine and loratadine on rhinovirus-induced intercellular adhesion molecule 1 upregulation and promoter activation in respiratory epithelial cells. *J Allergy Clin Immunol* 2001; 108: 221–228.
128. Fasce L, Ciprandi G, Pronzato C, *et al.* Cetirizine reduces ICAM-I on epithelial cells during nasal minimal persistent inflammation in asymptomatic children with mite-allergic asthma. *Int Arch Allergy Immunol* 1996; 109: 272–276.
129. De Sutter AIM, Saraswat A, van Driel ML. Antihistamines for the common cold. *Cochrane Database Syst Rev* 2015; 11: CD009345.
130. Crotta S, Davidson S, Mahlakoiv T, *et al.* Type I and type III interferons drive redundant amplification loops to induce a transcriptional signature in influenza-infected airway epithelia. *PLoS Pathog* 2013; 9: e1003773.
131. Iikura K, Katsunuma T, Saika S, *et al.* Peripheral blood mononuclear cells from patients with bronchial asthma show impaired innate immune responses to rhinovirus *in vitro*. *Int Arch Allergy Immunol* 2011; 155: Suppl. 1, 27–33.
132. Takaoka A, Hayakawa S, Yanai H, *et al.* Integration of interferon-α/β signalling to p53 responses in tumour suppression and antiviral defence. *Nature* 2003; 424: 516–523.
133. Khaitov MR, Laza-Stanca V, Edwards MR, *et al.* Respiratory virus induction of alpha-, beta- and lambda-interferons in bronchial epithelial cells and peripheral blood mononuclear cells. *Allergy* 2009; 64: 375–386.
134. Bosco A, Ehteshami S, Panyala S, *et al.* Interferon regulatory factor 7 is a major hub connecting interferon-mediated responses in virus-induced asthma exacerbations *in vivo*. *J Allergy Clin Immunol* 2012; 129: 88–94.
135. Sato M, Suemori H, Hata N, *et al.* Distinct and essential roles of transcription factors IRF-3 and IRF-7 in response to viruses for IFN-α/β gene induction. *Immunity* 2000; 13: 539–548.
136. Contoli M, Message SD, Laza-stanca V, *et al.* Role of deficient type III interferon-λ production in asthma exacerbations. *Nat Med* 2006; 12: 1023–1026.
137. Lopez-Souza N, Favoreto S, Wong H, *et al.* *In vitro* susceptibility to rhinovirus infection is greater for bronchial than for nasal airway epithelial cells in human subjects. *J Allergy Clin Immunol* 2009; 123: 1384–1390.e2.
138. Bochkov YA, Hanson KM, Keles S, *et al.* Rhinovirus-induced modulation of gene expression in bronchial epithelial cells from subjects with asthma. *Mucosal Immunol* 2010; 3: 69–80.
139. Sykes A, Edwards MR, Macintyre J, *et al.* Rhinovirus 16-induced IFN-α and IFN-β are deficient in bronchoalveolar lavage cells in asthmatic patients. *J Allergy Clin Immunol* 2012; 129: 1506–1514.e6.
140. Rochlitzer S, Hoymann H-G, Müller M, *et al.* No exacerbation but impaired anti-viral mechanisms in a rhinovirus-chronic allergic asthma mouse model. *Clin Sci (Lond)* 2014; 126: 55–65.
141. Kaiko GE, Loh Z, Spann K, *et al.* Toll-like receptor 7 gene deficiency and early-life *Pneumovirus* infection interact to predispose toward the development of asthma-like pathology in mice. *J Allergy Clin Immunol* 2013; 131: 1331–1339.e10.
142. Barclay WS, al-Nakib W, Higgins PG, *et al.* The time course of the humoral immune response to rhinovirus infection. *Epidemiol Infect* 1989; 103: 659–669.
143. Niespodziana K, Cabauatan CR, Jackson DJ, *et al.* Rhinovirus-induced VP1-specific antibodies are group-specific and associated with severity of respiratory symptoms. *EBioMedicine* 2015; 2: 64–70.
144. Alper CM, Doyle WJ, Skoner DP, *et al.* Prechallenge antibodies moderate disease expression in adults experimentally exposed to rhinovirus strain Hanks. *Clin Infect Dis* 1998; 27: 119–128.
145. Iwasaki J, Smith WA, Stone SR, *et al.* Species-specific and cross-reactive IgG1 antibody binding to viral capsid protein 1 (VP1) antigens of human rhinovirus species A, B and C. *PLoS One* 2013; 8: 1–11.
146. Iwasaki J, Smith W-A, Khoo S-K, *et al.* Comparison of rhinovirus antibody titers in children with asthma exacerbations and species-specific rhinovirus infection. *J Allergy Clin Immunol* 2014; 134: 25–32.
147. Heymann PW, Carper HT, Murphy DD, *et al.* Viral infections in relation to age, atopy, and season of admission among children hospitalized for wheezing. *J Allergy Clin Immunol* 2004; 114: 239–247.

148. Barends M, Van Oosten M, De Rond CGH, *et al.* Timing of infection and prior immunization with respiratory syncytial virus (RSV) in RSV-enhanced allergic inflammation. *J Infect Dis* 2004; 189: 1866–1872.
149. Stein RT, Sherrill D, Morgan WJ, *et al.* Respiratory syncytial virus in early life and risk of wheeze and allergy by age 13 years. *Lancet* 1999; 354: 541–545.
150. Welliver RC, Duffy L. The relationship of RSV-specific immunoglobulin E antibody responses in infancy, recurrent wheezing, and pulmonary function at age 7–8 years. *Pediatr Pulmonol* 1993; 15: 19–27.
151. Kusel MMH, de Klerk NH, Kebadze T, *et al.* Early-life respiratory viral infections, atopic sensitization, and risk of subsequent development of persistent asthma. *J Allergy Clin Immunol* 2007; 119: 1105–1110.
152. Jackson DJ, Gangnon RE, Evans MD, *et al.* Wheezing rhinovirus illnesses in early life predict asthma development in high-risk children. *Am J Respir Crit Care Med* 2008; 178: 667–672.
153. Koponen P, Helminen M, Paassilta M, *et al.* Preschool asthma after bronchiolitis in infancy. *Eur Respir J* 2012; 39: 76–80.
154. Lemanske RF, Dick EC, Swenson CA, *et al.* Rhinovirus upper respiratory infection increases airway hyperreactivity and late asthmatic reactions. *J Clin Invest* 1989; 83: 1–10.
155. Calhoun WJ, Dick EC, Schwartz LB, *et al.* A common cold virus, rhinovirus 16, potentiates airway inflammation after segmental antigen bronchoprovocation in allergic subjects. *J Clin Invest* 1994; 94: 2200–2208.
156. Calhoun WJ, Swenson CA, Dick EC, *et al.* Experimental rhinovirus 16 infection potentiates histamine release after antigen bronchoprovocation in allergic subjects. *Am Rev Respir Dis* 1991; 144: 1267–1273.
157. Moffatt MF, Kabesch M, Liang L, *et al.* Genetic variants regulating *ORMDL3* expression contribute to the risk of childhood asthma. *Nature* 2007; 448: 470–473.
158. Granell R, Henderson AJ, Timpson N, *et al.* Examination of the relationship between variation at 17q21 and childhood wheeze phenotypes. *J Allergy Clin Immunol* 2013; 131: 685–694.
159. Halapi E, Gudbjartsson DF, Jonsdottir GM, *et al.* A sequence variant on 17q21 is associated with age at onset and severity of asthma. *Eur J Hum Genet* 2010; 18: 902–908.
160. Calışkan M, Bochkov YA, Kreiner-Møller E, *et al.* Rhinovirus wheezing illness and genetic risk of childhood-onset asthma. *N Engl J Med* 2013; 368: 1398–1407.
161. Ono JG, Worgall TS, Worgall S. 17q21 locus and ORMDL3: an increased risk for childhood asthma. *Pediatr Res* 2014; 75: 165–170.

Disclosures: None declared.

Other titles in the series

ERS Monograph 71 – Idiopathic Pulmonary Fibrosis
Ulrich Costabel, Bruno Crestani and Athol U. Wells

ERS Monograph 70 – Imaging
R. Graham Barr, David G. Parr and Jens Vogel-Claussen

ERS Monograph 69 – Controversies in COPD
Antonio Anzueto, Yvonne Heijdra and John R. Hurst

ERS Monograph 68 – Lung Cancer
Anne-Marie C. Dingemans, Martin Reck and Virginie Westeel

ERS Monograph 67 – Obstructive Sleep Apnoea
Ferran Barbé and Jean-Louis Pépin

ERS Monograph 66 – Pulmonary Complications of HIV
Charles Feldman, Eva Polverino and Julio A. Ramirez

ERS Monograph 65 – Respiratory Epidemiology
Isabella Annesi-Maesano, Bo Lundbäck and Giovanni Viegi

ERS Monograph 64 – Cystic Fibrosis
Marcus A. Mall and J. Stuart Elborn

ERS Monograph 63 – Community-Acquired Pneumonia
James D. Chalmers, Mathias W. Pletz and Stefano Aliberti

ERS Monograph 62 – Outcomes in Clinical Trials
Martin Kolb and Claus F. Vogelmeier

ERS Monograph 61 – Complex Pleuropulmonary Infections
Gernot Rohde and Dragan Subotic